Indigenous Communalism

============

Indigenous Communalism

Belonging, Healthy Communities,
and Decolonizing the Collective

CAROLYN SMITH-MORRIS

RUTGERS UNIVERSITY PRESS
NEW BRUNSWICK, CAMDEN, AND NEWARK,
NEW JERSEY, AND LONDON

Library of Congress Cataloging-in-Publication Number: 2019002221

A British Cataloging-in-Publication record for this book is available from the British Library.

♾ The paper used in this publication meets the requirements of the American National Standard for Information Sciences—Permanence of Paper for Printed Library Materials, ANSI Z39.48–1992.

www.rutgersuniversitypress.org

Manufactured in the United States of America

In memory of my mom

In memory of my mom

Contents

Contents

Preface

Cylinders of cigarette ash lay corralled near the edge of the kitchen table, camouflaged in the flowers of the vinyl tablecloth. Whenever another truncated branch was shaken loose and fell, shattering among the swirling carnations and peonies, Ray just brushed it into the pile with his left pinky. Ray Keed was a six-foot-two elder among the Wiradjuri Aborigines of western New South Wales, Australia. In his generally quiet and sometimes stern way of moving about the world, he managed the affairs of his family, attended to his passionate and politically savvy wife, and chaired the Bogan River Wiradjuri Traditional Owners group. He took very seriously the work of shepherding in the next generation of leaders—whether his own Aboriginal kin or the string of non-Kooris (that is, non-Aboriginal) students brought to him by an anthropology professor from Sydney who'd worked with the Wiradjuri for many years. I was one in the string.

Ray and his wife, Valda, would be my hosts and supervisors for a summer's work on a Native Title claim. That is to say, they would house and feed me, introduce me to dozens of their Wiradjuri family and community members, lead me into conversations about culture, heritage, and tradition, and guide me away from inappropriate or offensive mistakes typical of non-Kooris. Our shared purpose was to document the many ways these people envisioned themselves as Wiradjuri, as belonging to a parcel of land, and as sharing a heritage that others did not share. Our relationship was quite (though not completely)[1] new when we did this work, but the intimacy of the topic was so personal that our bonds grew quickly.

It was in the early years after the passage of the Native Title Act, which made possible the first-ever claims to unalienated Crown land by Aboriginal entities, that Ray and Valda called me back to Australia. Through my mentor, Dr. Gaynor Macdonald at the University of Sydney, I was asked to help with the job of collecting and documenting the Bogan River Wiradjuri claim to one small claimable area. It was the mid-1990s, and I would live and work with Ray and Valda for several weeks gathering genealogies, family histories, place histories, and other data called for by the Act.

Because Ray and Valda were subtle and intelligent observers, they knew before my arrival all the ways I would reveal myself to be an outsider and in what ways I might be helpful. They had worked before with Gubba (white) younglings, trying to share with them the lessons of cultural difference, if not also of contemporary Aboriginal life. In fact, this work involved hours and hours of elders' talk, of which much came from Ray and Valda, but also passing time in the countryside and ancestral sites.

Our work was conducted around kitchen tables, on porch chairs, and while tending children. We laughed at stories that family members and Koori neighbors and friends told about their youth and the big family gatherings over their lifetimes. There were plenty of stories about conflicts between community members, but many more about the lifelong bonds within the community and the chronicles of sharing and care that sustained those relationships (see, e.g., Powell and Macdonald 2001). We even had a picnic at a site underneath 150-year-old rock paintings where we practiced throwing some boomerangs made by one of the cousins.

On my first night in their home for this job, Ray, Valda, and I reminisced about having met when I was an undergraduate student, and about the many undergraduates they had known. Ray and Valda took a group of students on a campout into the bush one time, also orchestrated by my mentor, Gaynor. Young visitors journeyed to this landscape of gum trees and brush flowers, where rabbits are a menace and the roadkill is kangaroos, and learned from these campouts about respect for the earth's resources, living more simply and with fewer commodities, and the Koori way of getting along with others, which they called "caring and sharing" (Macdonald 2000, 2017, forthcoming).

One night they told me about the time a big row erupted at the campsite over the washing of dishes. Rather than scraping the plates clean, using sparse liquid soap, and dunking all the dishes into a single pan of clean water to rinse, the Gubba kids were running the spigot for ten or fifteen minutes just to get the dishes clean. To Ray and Valda, such a wasting of water was not only an economic offense but a spiritual one. Australia is an extremely arid environment, with very few perennial sources of water. The Wiradjuri territory includes three seasonal rivers and lies generally north of the perennial Murray River, giving them relative water security. But this limited security is never taken for granted. Life is designed around those sources, and waterways are vital to local cultures, both practically and spiritually. The argument over water between Ray and those students embittered a few people but was a worthwhile and fundamental lesson about survival in Wiradjuri territory—not just about physical survival in an arid environment, but about spiritual and cultural survival in the context of presumptuous and privileged Others. Ray and Valda told this story to me on my first night in charge of washing up in their kitchen. I took the hint and let the dishes dry a little soapy.

Other good Gubba villains were teens who preened and flirted with each other too much, who ignored the wisdom of tradition and elders, or who were too often simply rude in expecting things to be like home. For professors who take students into foreign cultures, these are common enough lessons. But since I had come together with Ray and Valda not just as elders and young adult but as claimants and a research assistant, the lessons and stories took on greater dimensions.

In the highly political experience of a legal land claim, Indigenous peoples are made the subjects of intensive, outsider scrutiny. They have to prove the depth and duration of their cultural heritage in ways that dominant whites never do. What might have been family chatter or funny storytelling on another occasion was now being audio-recorded and added to the legal case file. Stories became accounts, family memories became Koori culture. I tried not to make the recording of these stories too obvious or intrusive and sometimes waited until I was alone to write things down. But the very fact that an anthropologist is taking notes on the conversation, turning it into a performance of ethnicity, is enough to make anyone a bit more philosophical and moralistic.[2]

A claim to Native Title for Aboriginal peoples in Australia is a momentous communal undertaking. It is a legal claim to ancestral lands made on the strength of demonstrated cultural affiliation with that land by a still-vibrant community. In fact, the very existence of a law allowing such claims for Native Title is a remarkable and relatively recent development. While some colonizing powers of the seventeenth and eighteenth centuries did their victims the courtesy of acknowledging them as (at least) human before taking their land, this was not the case in Australia.

Australian colonizers claimed the continent to be *terra nulius*, owned by no one and therefore "discoverable by a European nation which, by the simple act of effective possession, became the sovereign" (Wilkie 1985, 2).[3] No treaties were written, no arrangements were made regarding the relationship of Aboriginal peoples to the new government. Aboriginal people were invisible in the law, treated as feral pests in the landscape. Even as late as 1971, that eighteenth-century proclamation was reaffirmed: the famous Gove Land Rights Case declared again that Australia had been terra nulius when the Europeans arrived. So when the Native Title Act of 1993 was passed, although it was not an overwhelming victory for Aboriginal rights, people became hopeful that a new era for Australia was dawning.

So Ray and Valda told me their stories. One of the first stories Ray told me was about why geese fly in a V formation. It is, as readers well know, to help each other. Ray said each takes the lead, bearing the brunt of the wind for a period,

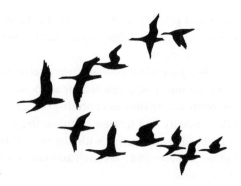

Figure 1. Geese flying in v-formation

then drops back to rest. Ray also described how, when one is shot or falls to the ground, two others drop with it, staying until it dies or gets well. Only then will they fly on together to reunite with their flock. Ray had witnessed this.

It was not so much this story as Ray's earnestness in telling it that left an impression with me. When an anthropologist is told a story by a new acquaintance, she can choose between a number of responses. Professionally she might record the content of the story or the manner or context in which it was told. Interpersonally she might focus on the correct performance of appreciation for the story, establishing her role as a respectful and engaged listener or demonstrating cultural competency to laugh, respond seriously, or make a retort or amendment. When Ray told me this story, we were driving to a small hill, formerly the dump site of a nearby mine, where Ray had lived as a child before his family got a house in Peak Hill. The gravity of that visit was clear in Ray's voice; he held fond memories of a happy childhood, but the wisdom and clarity of adulthood shadowed his memories with the racism and exclusions of colonialism. So his selection of that particular anecdote conveyed to me the priority that Ray hoped to emphasize. Valued community members are cared for throughout life, even when they falter.

In a small way, this form of caring would apply even to me, an American twentysomething more eager than skilled, but a trusted and years-long friend of this family. When help was needed and neither my mentor nor other locals were available to help, Ray and Valda called upon someone they already knew and trusted, despite the extra cost of an international plane ticket. That decision spoke volumes to me and was the first inspiration for this book.

In the weeks ahead, Ray, Valda, and their community made one lesson plain. Culture was not their lap-lap clothing or their rock art but an elaborated set of shared investments. Their heritage lay in their community, not solely in their land or any other material item. The most important traditions were ones remembered and kept alive by people committed to them. Though other details may vary, it is the working together on community-wide goals and the active repression and tamping down of selfish motives that allows a community as a whole to be sustained and a culture preserved. This was my first and most important lesson about the Wiradjuri, told through geese, and Ray wanted it on the record.

The second lesson was this: while communalist forces glue people together, the cohesion doesn't come without resistance. Managing individuals' normal but selfish motives is a main project of society, as Rousseau and other philosophers have argued. We have learned that our community benefits us and that we have to nourish it to survive. In my experience, native peoples do this better than most others, but there will always be conflict and diversity in how communal and individual motives are managed. And although I know you've heard this one too, Ray told this story:

> Two men go crawfishing—one black, one white. Each one catches two buckets of crayfish, and they're bringing 'em home. On the way, they come to a place where they have to walk across this log to get to the other side of a gorge. Blackfella walks across no problem. Whitefella crosses, losing half his crayfish. The whitefella asks the blackfella how he could cross without his crayfish jumping out of the buckets, to which the blackfella replies, "My crayfish are black crayfish. When one tries to get out, one of the others pulls him back down."

Thus began a career-long study of community building, with lessons of geese and crayfish. In the pages ahead, as in my career, these foundational lessons from the Wiradjuri give way to the Akimel O'odham of southern Arizona where my later work has been performed. The common threads between these two groups—of belonging, of generating "good" members of community, and of representing Indigenous perspective(s) in respectful and genuine ways—are what I convey in the pages ahead.

::::::::::

This book is not an ethnography of the Wiradjuri, though I relate Ray and Valda Keed's lessons here as an important backdrop to my work. This book is focused on my ethnographic work among the Akimel O'odham or Pima, to whom my work turned in graduate school.

As a non-Indigenous anthropologist, I view this book as an example of what Hale calls "cultural critique as ethnographic writing and theory building" (2006, 103). I am personally aligned with Indigenous struggles for self-determination, but my work and methodologies are only sometimes collaborative and co-owned with Indigenous people. This book clearly splits my "dual loyalties" (Hale 2006, 100) in favor of intellectual production, although it represents an advance on my previous efforts by further deconstructing a central ideological frame used with other Indigenous peoples.[4] More specifically, I address the authoritative bias that written texts about communalism, both generally and specific to Indigenous peoples, are given in Western systems of knowledge and law. My call for greater

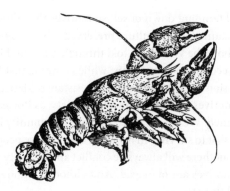

Figure 2. The not-so-
cooperative crayfish

attention to communalism is itself a form of deconstructive scrutiny that I hope
supports the Indigenous self-determinative imagination.

Since I awakened as an anthropologist within the native title and Indigenous
rights movements in New South Wales, I view this book as a project in recording evidence. I do not claim any contribution to that movement. Nor was I
involved in the generations-long Pima water claim battles. But it was in meetings with Peak Hill Wiradjuri about their community that I developed the perspective of this book. So the history and struggles of both tribes undergird the
rest of this book. I provide an overview of the Pima in my introduction, but the
Wiradjuri history is equally influential, so I briefly acknowledge it here. The Wiradjuri are, broadly defined, the Aboriginal people of a territory in New South Wales
containing three rivers: the Murrumbidgee, the Lachlan, and most of the Macquarie (Powell and Macdonald 2001, 2). The name encompasses a diversity of
local communities, each with its own autonomy and identity, but these communities have maintained active social and political networks both before the
Mission Period in Australia and since. Colonization of Wiradjuri country in the
1820s saw the arrival of livestock and the clearing and plowing of the landscape.
By the 1840s, most Aboriginal people used mission (or "pastoral") stations for
temporary or long-term camps, both for safety and for work.

The Bulgandramine Mission, fourteen miles northwest of the town of Peak
Hill, was home to Ray and Valda's families and many other Wiradjuri families
living in Peak Hill until 1941. It was Ray's sister-in-law, Rita Keed, who compiled
a book titled *Memories of Bulgandramine Mission*, with narratives and photos
about mission life, as local memories of it were failing. In it, she described the
mission as a "new kind of stability" over their former lives of conflict, warfare,
and flight, one that "enabled people to come to terms with their colonisers . . .
and to build relationships with the people who now controlled their livelihoods"
(1985, 6). The community that shared time at the Bulgandramine Mission and
the relationships developed there are remembered warmly, even reverently. This
includes relationships with whites. These memories are carried into the present

through the very various surnames adopted from white property owners by Wiradjuri ancestors of this area.[5]

When the mission abruptly closed and the Kooris were forced to find new places to live, many moved to camp closer to Peak Hill (Macdonald 2005). One spot in particular was the first field site I visited, the Dumps, where refuse and tailings from the nearby open-pit gold mine were discarded. Home to as many as two hundred Kooris for many years in the 1940s and 1950s (Powell and Macdonald 2001, 33), the Dumps, as well as the sites called Top Hill and Bottom Hill, were shack encampments built from flattened tin containers and other scraps. They were cold and lacked water and waste removal, leaving the Aboriginal people to manage these problems of a sedentary lifestyle without assistance. By the late 1950s, mounting complaints from both Aboriginal people and white Peak Hill residents about the substandard conditions led to state action, and housing in the town was slowly made available for Kooris. Though many were reluctant to leave the close-knit existence they shared in these multigenerational encampments, Aboriginal families began moving into town. They received single-family houses dispersed around Peak Hill. While the homes were a welcome comfort, the loss of community was deeply felt and remembered.

It is little wonder that the children born on the Bulgandramine Mission and at the Dumps, Top Hill, and Bottom Hill would become lifelong advocates for Aboriginal rights to these areas. This group included Ray and Valda Keed and many others with whom I worked in Peak Hill. Although I met the Peak Hill mob in 1986, soon after the Act had passed, it was not until 1995 that their own Native Title claim gave me the opportunity to return to and work in Peak Hill.[6]

As I mentioned, it was under Dr. Macdonald's direction and the guiding presence of Ray and Valda that I collected family trees, pictures, and narratives of life at the Dumps, Peak Hill, Bulgandramine, and other sites of work and home all over Wiradjuri country. We visited relatives and old friends in towns such as Dubbo, Wellington, and Cowra. We also toured sites in and around the claim, including the Dumps. In every important way, I was born as an anthropologist during this work and on that important site.

When I last left Peak Hill, there was still much to do on the Native Title claim. The Peak Hill Local Aboriginal Land Council now owns several businesses within the town. And Peak Hill itself is still filled with familiar names: Powells, Towneys, and Keeds. Their oft-repeated priority of "caring and sharing," instilled as a moral code from an early age, lies at the core of their ideas of being a good person.[7] Wiradjuri "caring and sharing" demand regular attention and time with each other. These closely held values are greatest, and often more visible, for those who grow up in such overtly communal settings, making them ideal case studies for community building. But as the events and narratives in this book show, communal values are part of every human society.

Indigenous Communalism

============

==============

Introduction

The global battle between individual rights and communal rights is reaching new levels of intensity and visibility. Consider three cases. The U.S. Affordable Care Act faced its greatest criticisms over the individual mandate, the legal requirement that most adults in the country purchase health insurance regardless of their current need or desire to do so. Political asylum cases are arbitrated in the international public media, like the Gambian woman who pled asylum in the United Kingdom to save her three-year-old daughter the suffering and risks of traditional genital cutting ceremony. (She was denied and deported along with her toddler.) And the global Indigenous movement, which after nearly a century of continuous, intergenerational efforts achieved the milestone Declaration on the Rights of Indigenous Peoples in 2007. In each of these emotionally and culturally charged cases, the interests of the individual are pitted directly against those of the community. And problematically, both the *community's* right to set each of these standards and each *individual's* right to flee them are protected under international doctrine. Cases like mandatory health insurance and female genital cutting seem to suggest that the West's radical and culturally dominant individualism—believed by many to be a requisite for modern humanitarian ethics—is losing ground.

This is the push-me-pull-you of individualism and communalism forever present in all human communities, throughout time. Around the world, cheap and ubiquitous forms of communication germinate new communities and communal expression never before possible, challenging our old definitions of "culture" and of cultural or communal rights. We now have a global community establishing itself in endless new ways while globalized groups within nations insist on new but common priorities of the group over individuals. Access to the internet, mass transportation, and twenty-four-hour news cycles foster these new moments and forms of tension, as Arjun Appadurai has been arguing since the

1970s. In response, individuals may feel homogenized culturally, their autonomy threatened, their rights abridged or never truly acknowledged. The specific global circumstances may be new, but the tension is actually millennia old: human society demands a constant balancing between individual and communal needs.

A focus on communalism as both a relational process and a moral engagement will decenter traditional subjects of Indigenous ethnographies. My focus is neither on identity, sovereignty, or self-determination nor on the traditional anthropological categories of study, such as religion, language, political system, or other major institutions of society. Instead, this book gives support to what Amit and Rapport (2002) intended in *The Trouble with Community*—for scholars to respect the processual and relational information that has been conveyed through ethnographic research among communal groups. Ultimately, I argue that individualism and communalism are better conceived as values upon which all humans draw than as taxonomic categories for entire groups of people.

Learning from Indigenous Peoples

Indigenous groups are unique as a category and practice many vibrant patterns of communalism. Despite decades of work by the UN Permanent Forum on Indigenous Affairs and its predecessor groups, no definition of "Indigenous peoples" was established, but an "understanding of the term" listed the following features:

- Self-identification and belonging
- Historical continuity and generation of new members over time
- The presence of, and the ability to represent for others, strong links to distinct territories, resources, social and cultural practices, and economic and political systems
- The resolve to maintain and reproduce their distinctive ways of life

These tenets operationalize a framework that gives political-economic legitimacy to groups who enjoyed "prior self-governance" (Bowen 2000). In this way, the term "Indigenous" becomes not a genetic litmus test or a blood and soil argument but a justification based in temporal durability, group self-determination, and communal survival, adaptation, and change.

In this ethnography of communalism, I illustrate each of these tenets as they speak to longevity and relationality in Pima (Akimel O'odham) Indian communalism. The frame of communalism indicates how important flexibility will be to the preservation of Indigenous lifeways into the future. I also emphasize how intergenerational longevity and relationality—as well as four specific processes of communalism—yield uniquely Indigenous communities. And in doing so, communalism is recognized as a value system among all humans, but at the center of Indigenous survival.

For illustrating how communalism is a vibrant and universal human process, Indigenous groups are powerful models. Inside this framing, the communalist meanings, relations, and mechanisms of culture appear both balanced and functional. They have long-term stability and adaptiveness to so much change and conflict. But in suggesting that there is global relevance in native strategies of community building and communalism, my goal is neither to enshrine Indigenous models behind a diorama glass nor to suggest that all human communities can perform or achieve what Indigenous peoples do. Put simply, communalism is a value system accessible by and to some extent practiced by all humans. Major differences lie in how much emphasis a community places on the group and how much and what types of freedom are retained by individuals.

Of several recent treatises on global Indigenous rights and of the activism and struggles of various native communities to achieve and enact their sovereignty, there is uniformity only in calls to respect local difference. In my ethnography of communalism, I too am providing "located and locatable voices" (Waitere and Allen 2011, 48). Accordingly, I must stress that in my frame of these lessons as "Indigenous communalism," I attempt neither to homogenize the experience of indigeneity nor to suggest that native peoples face globalization in the same ways worldwide. That struggle continues in diverse ways (Stewart-Harawira 2005). My intention is to capture and record what I have recognized as shared values among Indigenous peoples but that are admittedly present across human groups globally in different forms. In the concluding chapter I rely on a number of other scholars' writings and activists' work to consider Indigenous communalism in this global context.

COMMUNALISM IN THE GLOBAL INDUSTRIAL COMPLEX

At a most general level, communalism is about community building or the creation of community. But in the millennia of mass mobility and transnationalism, the referential capacity of the word "community" has exploded. For any study of *a* community, there exists a danger in identification of too large or amorphous a group. Similarly, use of preexisting assumptions—for example, that a given Indian reservation naturally constitutes a complete and cohesive community—may also be inappropriate (Smith-Morris 2006a). The study of "community" could, therefore, encompass a vast intellectual space across the social sciences and Indigenous studies, from semiotic and identity studies to the more material questions of sharing, reciprocity, and cooperation.

Theorists from human behavioral ecology (HBE) have given us some compelling, and sometimes surprising, evidentiary estimates of what happens among human groups as they attempt to survive in groups. They can estimate, for example, how often and under what circumstances individuals will forgo personal benefits in favor of a perceived or real group benefit. It is surprisingly often, under certain circumstances. Overall, they find plenty of self-interest in group actions since the success of a sharing and cooperative group helps all of its members; but HBE theorists also recognize self-interested altruism as a communalist tendency and therefore help us envision what communalism looks like. By engaging a definition of communalism not as a sociopolitical type but as a set of moral priorities or values, we can both recognize the long-term benefits of cooperation and push even further into the biobehavioral studies of our adapted minds and even into the interpretive work of moral anthropology.

::::::::::

But for most of the Akimel O'odham with whom I worked in my research, the notion of community is not a resource to be manipulated, as theories of social capital and behavioral ecology abstractly suggest.[1] Nor do the relationships around which their lives are built conform neatly to cost-benefit or energy allocation analyses. They are complicated by personal and community history, taking on new meanings with every need, challenge, and success. Native forms of community, not unlike any other community that shares a history of trauma, are heavily colored by the racialized injustice and overpowering capitalist and antienvironmental influence. So while academic and scientific explanations have their place and utility, community for natives is inescapably a moral question.[2]

Action and applied research would form yet another sector studying community and communalism, measuring and harnessing the power of community for particular ends. And there are economic, business, and development agendas that hinge on notions of what makes a community successful or healthy. Fueled by campaigns to privatize and decentralize global development campaigns, and guided by research into things like social capital, participatory methods, and community engagement, community building is now a "fundable project."[3] And finally, community is an essential metric for political engagement and "sustainable" development, both of which are now recognized as human rights.[4] In short, the study of community and communalism encompasses all facets of group life—from social capital and community empowerment to human behavioral ecology (Smith-Morris 2006a, 2006b; Manderson 2010; Cohen 1999; Amit 2002a, 2002b; Amit and Rapport 2002).

::::::::::

Accordingly, this book takes up broad questions of cultural values. How do cultures build up around communal and cooperative priorities? How do they maintain their communal ideals in the face of long and continuing colonial influence? I am particularly concerned with dismantling the binary assumptions still regnant in global discourses. Anthropologists like the "generalized lumps" of individualism or communalism, undifferentiated either within or between themselves (Kusserow 2004, v). Those value binaries that have inspired many from Weber to Hofstede have not served me well in my field sites.[5] This book illustrates why and attempts a remedy.

If we look at the "webs of social relations that encompass shared meanings and above all shared values" (Etzioni 1998, xiii), we achieve a view of community as process, not as cultural construct or as a structure containing a given set of features. In the tradition illuminated by Marilyn Strathern, Carol Gilligan, Jeffrey Cohen, Carol Stack, and Rhoda Halperin, my work pays witness to the *process* of building relationships, engagement, and negotiation over time. For my purposes, the process of setting rules for good behavior and generating or enforcing conformity is a perpetual obligation, each individual member deciding rationally to remain part of that rule-guided community.[6] This book is therefore an inquiry into the everyday mechanisms that form community, of communalist decisions and actions, and of the capacities for change that allow communities to hold themselves together and thrive despite pressures of increasingly globalized forms of mobility, market participation, and governance.

Finally, to understand communalism, we must consider the industrial settler state's scientific, legal, and programmatic obsession with individualism. Scholars and developers alike recognize that to build community requires individual investment. It is also easier and faster to motivate and incentivize individuals rather than whole communities en masse. But the field of "economic development" for native groups is littered with the corpses of individualist projects that failed to appreciate the role and importance of local moral structures oriented toward the group (see, e.g., Mosse 1997, 1999, 2006). What reformers of "development" (now "sustainable development") recognize is that, contrary to being ideologically opposed, the values of individualism and communalism are actually inseparable, a synergistic pair. Campaigns to promote community *must* harness individual motives if they are to succeed. Projects to build community rely upon, and must therefore generate, certain types of individuals to lead and remain committed to those projects. In short, the work of communalism is as much about the group as it is about the values and goals instilled in its individual members. The individual/communal binary is, therefore, taken up in several ways in the pages ahead.

The Politics of Indigeneity—Terms, Frames, and Representations

Many Indigenous authors and scholars alike have explained how Indigenous groups tend to identify themselves narrowly—by locality, language dialect, or kinship—in contrast to the homogenized categories developed by academics and still in use. For example, about the broad categorization of multiple O'odham groups under a single "Piman" nomenclature, Brenneman wrote, "The very notion of a 'Pimería Alta' places the O'odham within a European conceptual framework, implying a structural cohesiveness or unified organization that did not exist among the scattered, autonomous O'odham communities [prior to colonial era]" (2014, 207). Instead, this large swath of related but distinct groups was *represented* as unified because it was either easier or expedient for colonial authorities to do so. Frederick Hoxie (2008) described how academic experts have written about Native Americans and how beginning in the 1950s, formerly flat representations began to reflect deeper insights and native voices and perspectives. Nigel Rapport has similarly argued that anthropological definitions of culture have tended to be overly holistic and homogenizing and that such illusions are "worthless in contemporary existential contexts of hybridity (Bhabha) and creolisation (Hannerz), of synchronicity (Tambiah) and compression (Paine)" (Rapport 1997, 382; also see Rapport 2002). And others like Lee (2006), Conklin (Conklin and Graham 1995; Conklin 2002), and Ramos (1987, 1994, 1998) have argued that "Indigeneity" is itself a recent concept only, but vigorously debated and strategically employed. It is not just what Indigenous peoples say about themselves but what academics, activists, politicians, and the literati (all of which now include Indigenous persons) want that movement to be. I take up issues of representation in chapter 3 but must introduce several terms and frames here at the beginning.

Most contemporary scholars, especially non-Indigenous ones, have learned to step lightly around the question of exactly what is uniquely "Indigenous" and how this term might be defined. Despite decades of ethnographic, community-based, and even native-authored research into the specific and/or patterned characteristics of different Indigenous groups, we are loath to generalize. Even Indigenous activists can be either vague or noticeably high-level in their characterizations of this concept of primary importance. The concern, of course, is in creating a description that fails to faithfully represent all such groups globally. This definitional challenge was the focus of much of the work building up to the 2007 UN Declaration on the Rights of Indigenous Peoples (DRIP), the resulting definition from which I quote below. But first I review two satellite terms—namely "native" and "tribal"—because these also appear in the pages ahead.

The term "native" has at least two meanings. First, it is an indication of association with the country, region, or circumstances of one's birth. To this meaning, all people have rightful access, but I will give little attention to it in this volume. The second meaning indicates membership within the community known as Native Americans, whose precolonial natal origin is in the Americas but whose community membership now may be determined in broader ways than natal location. In the United States, some Indigenous persons have embraced the term "Native American" to refer to themselves and to their communities as peoples. Others across the North and South American continents certainly have not. Most Pimas with whom I have worked refer to themselves first as "Pima,"

"O'odham," or "Indian" in familiar circles and as "Native American" only in academic circles.

Anthropologists and activists have debated these terms for decades, but the material impacts of these debates have changed in important ways over the past century and especially in the past two or three decades. In a series of articles initiated with Adam Kuper's "The Return of the Native," *Current Anthropology* published a span of viewpoints from Indigenous and non-Indigenous authors (Kuper et al. 2003; Garrett 2003). Kuper's initial piece acknowledges the history of naming for peoples linked by their more "harmonious" existence with nature and by their shared history of having been colonized by imperial, industrialist powers. But he also raises the question of knowledge, myth, and history as authoritative sources for those who would name these peoples, sources that offer contradictory answer to questions such as this: "Who were the original people in a place?" Kuper also names as relevant for the global Indigenous movement the contemporary political boundaries under which one or more Indigenous peoples may be living and the implications of these political definitions for the distribution of resources, care, and legal protection.[7] I take up this semiotic and discursive landscape in a rather different way, examining ethnographic evidence of community building and avoiding the legalistic arguments. I realize this stops short of suggesting how my data and model may impact definitions of Indigeneity, and that is intentional.

As some of the authors in the *Current Anthropology* collection address, the term "native" can be especially problematic in light of colonial-era displacement, contemporary economic and political disenfranchisement, and voluntary diasporic and migratory movements. For example, Indigenous peoples do not relinquish their ties to ancestral and traditional territories though they may travel or migrate. So the restrictiveness of a natal origin litmus test is unacceptable for many. In short, being native to a place remains a relevant and respected source of Indigenous identity, but it is not a sufficient one.

On the other hand, Indigenous leaders firmly reject claims by non-Indigenous actors that "we are all Indigenous" and part of a global humanity (Kuper et al. 2003; Asch et al. 2004; Asch et al. 2006). They expose the privilege of those who *choose* when to be Indigenous and when to claim affiliation with a dominant ethnicity or nationhood. They further reject the trope of "ethnicity" as failing to address the uniqueness of Indigenous experience. That is, "ethnicity" is a nosological category into which minority groups of all kinds can be housed, contained, measured, and dehistoricized. Treating Indigenous peoples as minorities in their own homelands or among those who exercised a right of mobility fails to see the "residual of colonialism" that such nosologies enact (Sium, Desai, and Ritskes 2012, vii).

The second satellite term, "tribal," is used in this book in both rhetorical and anthropological ways. The anthropological label of "tribe" was historically reserved for groups with a certain pattern of subsistence, political organization, and size (Service 1971). It is also a term still commonly used in the United States to refer to Indigenous groups (although the northern New Mexican puebloans do not use "tribe" to describe themselves). My use is typically in reference to the Gila River Indian Community, since the word is still in use there. Furthermore, the term "tribal" also highlights "an alternative mode of identity and social behavior" (Brysk 2000, 1) and includes a sensitivity to nature and one's place within a local and planetary community. Once again, local specificity will be relied upon to promote clarity and respect in use of the term "tribal." When this fails, it helps to remember that the very discipline of anthropology originated in data from autochthonous communities, whom we described as "native" or "Indigenous" but also, for a time, as "savage" and "barbarian." Terms do and must change to address changing knowledge and circumstance.

Finally, the term "Indigenous" was the one chosen by the United Nations when it named a special working group in 1982 to address the unrecognized, stateless peoples already active and seeking recognition in that international domain. It was chosen over terms like "native," "primitive," and "Aboriginal" as a way of reconciling two dominant approaches to self-definition by cultural groups. The contentious "blood and soil" approach, which recognizes only native-born claims of recognition within a precise geographical coordinate, has an immobilizing impact both on state powers and within the diverse global community of Indigenous peoples. When pressed, I therefore defer to the United Nations Permanent Forum on Indigenous Issues for an understanding of the term "Indigenous":

> Considering the diversity of Indigenous peoples, an official definition of "Indigenous" has not been adopted by any UN-system body. Instead the system has developed a modern understanding of this term based on the following:
>
> - Self-identification as Indigenous peoples at the individual level and accepted by the community as their member
> - Historical continuity with pre-colonial and/or pre-settler societies
> - Strong link to territories and surrounding natural resources
> - Distinct social, economic or political systems
> - Distinct language, culture and beliefs
> - Form non-dominant groups of society
> - Resolve to maintain and reproduce their ancestral environments and systems as distinctive peoples and communities[8]

This multifaceted definition attempts to capture the diversity I have seen among native groups globally and goes a long way toward recognizing the community centeredness that I take as my subject.

Indigenous communalism deserves greater attention as part of the ideological decolonization begun last century and invigorated by the passage of the DRIP. Considering the limited financial and technological resources of so many Indigenous peoples since colonization, in contrast to the state and international governments and market institutions that might have opposed them, the passage of the DRIP was an astounding achievement. These rights could not be minority rights, which are conferred on an individual basis; the central role of the collectivity had to remain intact. The communalist agenda of the declaration gets at the heart of Indigenous identity, yet it is not so rigid as to envision Indigenous peoples at a single (historic) moment in time without a future. That it serves the "multiple patterns of human association and interdependency" (e.g., Muehlebach 2003) visible among the globe's Indigenous communities is testimony to its careful construction.

Why Is Communalism Missing?

And yet the term 'communalism' is noticeably absent from the DRIP definition. Clear and consistent evidence to the family (Guillory and Wolverton 2008; Michielutte et al. 1994) and community centeredness (Smith-Morris 2004, 2007; Overing and Passes 2002) of Indigenous communities is perhaps intended by the DRIP terms "historical continuity" and "ancestral," but it is far from clear. The existing definition leaves maximum flexibility to those postcolonial entities to determine their own cultural futures, which is a laudable solution. But in Barnard's (2006) words, the DRIP and any definition of "Indigenous" is a legal one, not an anthropological one. In other words, some of the key processes that sustain these communities—namely their commitment to each other and (specific for Indigenous peoples) to relational, ancestral, and sometimes place-based heritage—are left to the imagination. Some may see this as a protection, in that Indigenous peoples would not be restricted in their future work and self-determination; but there might also be vulnerabilities in a failure to recognize and protect communalist mechanisms. At a minimum, further consideration of the question seems warranted.

Corntassel is more precise on the issue of communal aspects of Indigeneity. He insists that peoplehood involves "the interlocking features of language, homeland, ceremonial cycles, and sacred living histories [such that] a disruption to any one of these threatens all aspects of everyday life" (2012, 89).[9] By adding this shared element of peoplehood to the territorial and place-based identity claims already covered in the DRIP definition, we approach a more complete treatment of what is uniquely Indigenous.

By preparing an ethnography of communalism, rather than one of a particular "community" or of a more traditional study of "political" organization, I have tried to capture these implied but vague elements of Indigeneity. If Native American scholarship and intellectual tradition are any indication, then survivance will indeed require the continuing commitment of Indigenous peoples to relational engagement with each other. Repeated in scientific and literary scripts about Indigenous groups is a continuing attitude toward "caring and sharing" (Macdonald 2000, 87), "aesthetics of conviviality" (Overing and Passes 2002), and community building. These social and affective attitudes are not simply practices but "ways of being" that contribute to a "generalised moral obligation" (Macdonald 2000, 88). The distinction follows Eric Wolf's (1982) retheorizing of "mode of production" not as an economic system for meeting subsistence needs but as a larger "set of social relations" defining how individuals engage with each other. For the Wiradjuri,

> Sharing requires a strong conception of personal autonomy and personal property because it is precisely in the nature of how one shares what one has rights over that one is, in turn, defined. Too much giving destroys a relationship: the power becomes too great to sustain sociality. . . . In addition, the more powerful person will need to sustain a certain quality of social interaction in order that people will want to continue to ask of them. Not to be asked reduces one's power accordingly. (Macdonald 2000, 95)

Although not explicit in her formulation, communal balance is also recognized by Stewart-Harawira (2005) as a patterned Indigenous characteristic. She suggests that Indigenous ways of "being in the world" (154) involve a number of elemental principles. These principles include the "profound interconnectedness of all existence"; that every individual "has its own unique life force"; a "deep obligation" of humans to guardianship for the earth and all life; a commitment to balance (expressed through reciprocity, which resonates with Macdonald's discussion of Wiradjuri "caring and sharing" above); and a dedication to compassion, "said to be the element most lacking in today's society" (Stewart-Harawira 2005, 156). The model I use to organize this ethnography respects each of these principles.

The Dangers of Universalism

As I have been careful to explain my approach to Indigenous peoples, I also acknowledge the immeasurable but important differences within the category of Indigenous: differences in political aims and histories, differences between those in "developed" and "developing" states, differences "between those struggling for sheer survival and those seeking forms of cultural, economic and political equality, recognition and restitution" (Corntassel 2012,, 251). I say more about these at various points, but overgeneralizing about Indigenous peoples rightfully inspires caution among scholars, activists, and the authors of the DRIP.

The latter, after all, refused to "define" the term "Indigenous" and offered only "a modern understanding of the term" (see inset quote above).

Why is there such firm disagreement between the antiuniversalists and those who insist that Indigenous ontologies do exist? Is there a way to talk about patterns among Indigenous peoples without slipping into racialized and racializing overgeneralizations? Sium, Desai, and Ritskes "firmly reject" the stance of a "Western styled humanism that proclaims "We are all Indigenous," conflating Indigeneity with humanity (2012, vi). The tension is perhaps best resolved by understanding these different ways of *being* as, instead, different and "highly situated" ways of knowing (Nygren 1999, 270). Such a view not only recognizes the very fundamental and uneasily changed orientations of a cultural group but also avoids racializing the difference. In this book I recognize humans for their universal *capacity* for communalism, respect for nature, family centeredness, and the rest, but I pay witness to undeniable variation across groups and to distinctive characteristics in Indigenous communalism.

Arguments over who or what is Indigenous may simply engage the wrong question. Many have found illuminating on this point Alan Barnard's comparison of the Kalahari revisionists and the Vienna school of anthropology. In brief, Barnard finds "there is no anthropological definition of 'Indigenous' that is unproblematic. It is a legal concept" (2006, 11). His argument mirrors Rapport's, that anthropologists need not choose between polarized attitudes toward Indigeneity but should instead evaluate local requirements for legitimate political goals related to the enjoyment of ancestral resources (Barnard 2006; see also Rapport 1998). I have never felt such tension over the special category of Indigeneity since the Indigenous peoples with whom I have lived and worked made such different choices and had such different forms of knowledge than my own. Accordingly, the model of communalism I illustrate here *could* be adapted for non-Indigenous groups, but the balance of values would be quite different. Indigenous peoples affirm communal change and adaptation, while non-Indigenous peoples are more likely to pursue individual goals, identities, and citizenship. The Indigenous balance of communalism and individualism (and it is a balance, not exclusively one or the other) therefore adds intergenerational (and sometimes place-based) priorities, which I am careful to specify throughout the volume.

It may be impossible to define "Indigenous" because it has proven nearly impossible to define "culture." In their general history and critical review of various definitions of "culture," Alfred Kroeber and Clyde Kluckhohn said that "if there be any single central tendency in the attempts to conceptualize culture over eighty years, it has been that of denying in principle a search for 'the' [single] factor" of culture(1952, 180). But taking seriously the premise that culture is a shared trait, then communalism—the valuing of the group *as* a group—is perhaps culture's only prerequisite. That is, whatever values, beliefs, and practices may appear, if we are to call them "cultural," they must be *shared* by a group of people who are actively relating to each other in some way. To some extent, all cultural groups must value themselves *as* a group.

One might argue that the postmodern turn in anthropology, during which academic definitions of culture transformed from more material to more meaning-centered frameworks, produced a corresponding reconsideration of this *shared* character in processes of meaning making. Take, for example, Clifford Geertz's definition of culture: "an historically transmitted pattern of meanings embodied in symbols, a system of inherited conceptions expressed in symbolic forms by means of which men communicate, perpetuate, and develop their knowledge about and their attitudes toward life" (1973, 356). The nouns in this definition, "pattern of meanings" and "system of conceptions," point to meanings, not materials, a major shift. The change represented a changing world, one in which the speed and breadth of culture contact and sharing demanded a more interactional sense of culture. As postmodern perspectives and forces of globalization have impacted the world and anthropological theory, cultural groups are now spoken of in more relativist terms.[10] What has remained the same is the idea that culture is communal, a process, something shared and transmitted through groups. This change in definition, and indeed our ability to shift to a new definition at all, is important for communal rights and for the survival of native peoples. Kenrick and Lewis summarize the more dynamic view that is taken up by most advocates and scholars of culture today: "[A] dynamic view of how culture is negotiated and transformed as it emerges in and between individuals in a particular place, rather than being a static body of unchanging values and practices to which and individual conforms" (2004, 6). Increasingly, then, both scholars of culture and activists working in defense of a particular cultural group must recognize not only the products of but also the processes by which collectivities of various kinds come to share values. This is a message echoed by the prolific and insightful Vered Amit, who says that communities can only be "truly felt and claimed by its potential members if they are able to realize it socially, in their relations and familiarity with some, if not every other constituent" (2002a, 8).

To be sure, the development of laws and declarations around collective rights raises new challenges for Indigenous peoples. I am thinking here of the new ways that "culture" and "Indigeneity" are mobilized and of conflicts between collective and individual rights, which I take up directly in chapter 6. But I also heed the warnings of Hodžić, Kuper, and others that we should be cautious of entering a rights versus culture debate. "Culture" can be mobilized in specific ways, both in support of local traditions and in support of state and modernist agendas. In her discussion of Ghana's domestic violence laws, Hodžić (2009, 348) described how "culture writ large has become the primary language of popular resistance to Western impositions, including the frameworks of human rights and liberalism" (see also Kuper et al. 2003, 395). She evaluated the place of community in colonial health and found it impossible to avoid the gendered impact of "rights" appeals because so many of the cultural practices requiring "liberation" had been focused on the bodies and sexuality of women: female circumcision/cutting, widow burning, women's veiling. But Hodžić also showed how politicians can use language to dress one idea in the mantle of an entirely different one. Individual, partner, family, and communal rights are all contested simultaneously in this case, but the term "culture" had been deployed only to protect "the family." And in Hodžić's estimation, not all members of the family were protected.

We seem to be developing keener eyesight for nonindividualist pressures, not only for Indigenous peoples but even in the most individualistic societies. But we still need better methods and tools for discerning communalism, its benefits and reasonable limits. Such tools will be valuable for Indigenous claims to sovereignty and land title, for questions of postcolonial reparations or reconciliation, and for peaceful coexistence.

Communalism and Health

The health focus of my own research will be most evident in chapter 5, "Asserting Communalism." Health and healing is just one of many realms of experience in which the connectedness of individuals is not only important but also given some attention by researchers and professionals in that realm. That is, doctors, nurses, and case managers are often aware of the social determinants of health and of the impact of isolation (or, alternatively, social support) on health and recovery from illness. It should not be surprising that the realm of health and healing therefore offers a substantial literature on community, social capital, and the social networks that define, facilitate, and work to improve health care.

Health and medicine in Indigenous and non-Western contexts provide a rich opportunity to contrast the assumptions of Western biomedicine, for considering the ideological basis of certain health care practices, and for evaluating the symbolic and intellectually colonizing effects of certain healing traditions. Where critical medical anthropology has drawn attention to the structural violence of colonial and postcolonial institutions (Anderson 2014; Farmer et al. 2004), we now have a clearer vision of peoples' vulnerabilities (Quesada, Hart, and Bourgois 2011) at the margin of those institutions, where cultural change (including changes in healing culture) impacts the many, integrated aspects of a community's life. For Indigenous peoples, the integration of Western biomedical healing traditions—for all its benefits—also brings with it cultural and ideological ideas that resist and can destroy communalist values.

For these reasons, one of the cases of communalism I feel I must address in this book—because it is a medical/health-related case of communal self-determination, though it is *not* common to Indigenous peoples—is female genital cutting (FC). Readers would misconstrue my discussion (in chapters 4 and 6) if they were to take it as a statement about Indigenous people. It is not. My discussion of FC is an explicit, and I believe necessary, conversation about the diversities of communalist practice. Specifically, that part of the discussion ahead questions our commitment to respecting communalism, and community self-determination, when the collective abridges individual human rights. Conflicts between individual and collective human rights are among the most inflammatory and emotional cases of our time, but they demand respectful, reasoned, and morally engaged responses.

The topic of communalism and health also draws upon important guidelines for research and care, including informed consent, consent for research, and ownership of knowledge. Enormous strides toward protection of human rights have been made in the past one hundred years in large part thanks to a respect for universal but individual human experience. That said, through deliberation over competing individual and collective goals in each of these same topics, I show how communalism in health remains a relevant concern.

Community with the Name "Gila River"

The Gila River Indian Community is home to the Akimel O'odham, or "River People" in their own language. They are commonly called Pima, likely a phonetic conflation of the O'odham phrase *pi'añi mac*, which means "I don't know" and was likely heard often by early visitors to O'odham territory (see Russell 1908). The Akimel O'odham were subsistence farmers long before the Spaniards arrived in the early nineteenth century and are descendants of the ancient Hohokam who resided here since about 400 CE (Bahti 1968; Fagan 2006).[11] They shared partnerships and kinship with the Tohono O'odham and the Hia'ced peoples to the west and south and trading relations in all directions.[12] They had more competitive and violent relationships with some of the Apaches to the east and north, in part because of their stable agriculture-based economy that gave them relative wealth for this region.

As early as the 1740s, the Akimel O'odham were producing surplus foods and are known to have shared and sometimes bartered these surpluses. DeJong describes the Pima as "well on the road to economic prosperity" by the end of the eighteenth century (2011, 9). But overwhelming numbers of white colonists moving to the area and the failure of the federal government to enforce promised legal protections led to near destruction of the Akimel O'odham livelihood by 1870. There were also periods of drought in this era, which produced several decades of famine and extreme poverty, dragging this once prosperous commu-

nity into the dependency, alcoholism, and other family and community trau-
mas that characterize so many North American tribes.[13] Today, thanks in part
to a 2004 landmark water-rights settlement, Pima agriculture has been revital-
ized. With income from other industry developments on the reservation,
including casino ventures, the Pima economy is improved and, with it, their
health, self-governance, and independence.

Much has been written about the historic expertise of Pima farmers (e.g., Russell 1903; Castetter and Bell 1942; Hackenberg 1962; Rea 1997; DeJong 2003).
Rather than review that history here, I point to only one social and cultural characteristic that sustained that subsistence strategy. Namely, farming demanded a
somewhat sedentary lifestyle and certain corresponding adaptations in cooperation.[14] Humans have adapted to cooperative social life in a variety of ways
throughout the evolution of our species, and the O'odham offer one example of
this process. In short, cooperative adaptations include the diversity of local skills,
preferences, and values that emerge and are sustained to promote a group's ability to thrive and "propel individual actions, decision-making, and behavior in
particular situations" (Henrich and Henrich 2007, 9). The Akimel O'odham's
location in the water-rich basin of the Gila River rewarded agricultural innovation. In turn, the regularity of successful food production reinforced local investments in irrigation ditches (which demands group labor) and shared defensive
strategies.

For the purposes of this book, we look not so much to cooperative agricultural economies as to the "content biases" toward cooperation that irrigation
agriculture produced—that is, the cultural tendencies toward ideas and elements
that "fit together in some cognitive or psychological sense" with cooperative agriculture (Henrich and Henrich 2007, 11). For example, the building of cooperative relationships, or relations of reciprocity, allowed the O'odham to identify
specific people (close kin first but also extended kin and eventually non-kin) on
whom they could rely for help. A second example of a cooperative "content bias"
is the evolution of social norms for prosociality, or being helpful to those viewed
as members of one's cultural group. At Wiradjuri, this was called "sharing and
caring" (Macdonald 2000). In the words of an Akimel O'odham father, the son
of a farmer, it is simply "being Indian."

The circumstances of my entry into the Gila River Indian Community speak
to the (reasonable) question of my authority on the topic of Indigenous communalism and cooperation. It was far different from my entry into the community
of Wiradjuri at Peak Hill (see the preface), where I had been invited and even
escorted into place by a trusted friend of the community. There, I was settled
securely into the warm and welcoming home of elders who held leadership positions in the Native Title claim on which I would work. I was given my own bed
and a family-like relationship with those supervisors, so my position vis-à-vis
the rest of the community was clear to everyone and I did not need to explain

my presence as we went about our work. At Gila River, on the other hand, I was a complete stranger. From my graduate school campus in Tucson, Arizona, I was surrounded by Indigenous groups in equally provocative circumstances. One morning in the Fall of 1996, I saw an advertisement posted on the student job bulletin board. The letterhead at the top of the ad showed a community seal, an easily recognized desert scene with saguaro cactus. The director of the Diabetes Education Center in a tribal hospital wanted to conduct some program evaluation in her department and needed a volunteer researcher to design and perform the work. The center was two hours away. This diabetes outcome study seemed custom-made for me, having held a job in hospital evaluation immediately before graduate school and still energized from my work on Wiradjuri Native Title. It combined native issues with my focus on health and health care, and I had a skill set in program evaluation that would be helpful to the tribe. Within a week, I was making my first visit to Sacaton, Arizona, the Gila River Indian Community's government seat.[15]

It was in the Gila River hospital, Hu Hu Kam Memorial, and through my volunteer work for the Diabetes Education Center there that I made my first friendships and formal contacts with the Akimel O'odham. My visits, once every two to four weeks for several years, started at the Diabetes Education Center and only slowly embraced wider circles of contacts and familiarity. For a time I was able to stay in the hospital housing, reserved for temporary medical students and clinical staff performing residencies in the tribal hospital. It was conveniently close to the hospital, but it was also strangely isolated, and even empty most of the nights I stayed there. So within a year I had developed friendships with Sacaton locals that were close enough to tolerate my request to sleep on their couch. Once this happened, my experience of Gila River transformed from visiting volunteer to anthropologist.[16]

The hospital is situated near the center of Sacaton, where the community's government offices are also located. Just a mile from the major interstate that transects the reservation, Sacaton is one of the most populous of the seven reservation districts stretching diagonally from the Pee-Posh farms in the northwest to Blackwater in the southeast. Sacaton had no gas station when I started volunteering there but has changed and grown substantially. New offices for the government were constructed and new buildings and programs added to Hu Hu Kam Memorial, which itself became part of the Gila River Health Care Corporation. New and better roads, upgraded parks, and more street lighting have also helped keep this small and quiet town vibrant in its distinctive and only moderately commoditized way.

Research for this book occurred over long periods of time and more than one project, in communities that have been in constant metamorphosis. The research questions have covered several topics: cultural change, health, foodways, and family life. But as for all cultural anthropology, the experiences of the people who offered me their narratives on any of these focal topics often meandered into other issues. The projects included the program evaluation mentioned above, in which I helped program staff assess the impact of diabetes education classes for pregnant women on birth outcomes. That project also served to introduce me to the structure and administration of Hu Hu Kam Memorial, to the Gila River Indian Community Council and its standing committee dedicated to health, and to O'odham staff in both organizations who would become my first friends in the community. My ethnography of diabetes in the community (outside of the hospital) required three years to set up and another three to complete but gave me more than a year full-time on the reservation. A third major project was a multiyear study of life stressors and their health impacts, a project that has involved O'odham collaborators and several students. Over a period of two decades, reservation life has revealed itself from many perspectives, always as a culturally vibrant, family-centered dynamic but with a generous supply of modernity's poverty, crime, work, food, and drugs. It was also in this period that the line between my professional and personal relationships sometimes blurred, as is often the case (if not the goal) for anthropologists. Never did this blurring make my O'odham informants vulnerable, but it did move the work into more personal space and my obligation to them into greater depths.

Finally, the ethnographic data have emerged not just from direct inquiries but through years of participant observation, direct study of multiple facets of community, and a perspective seasoned with both scholarly and personal engagement. My conclusions draw heavily from the interstitial spaces between project hypotheses. That is, the fundable research questions that sent me to the reservation were not the ones that captured the full spectrum of rich cultural information. And herein lies the importance of participant observation as a research methodology and a cornerstone of anthropological science. Only when I was free from tree-scale, hypothesis-driven data collection and able to record the broad variety of details that captured my attention and awe were the forest-scale patterns of culture apparent. Likewise, only after years of reflection across multiple projects and multiple communities have these pieces reached the critical mass and cohesiveness that warrant a monograph.

One of the things that distinguishes this discussion of native community building from others that are written about remote villages or subsistence economies is that both the Akimel O'odham and the Peak Hill Wiradjuri were both colonized generations ago and are now living deeply enmeshed within wage economies and industrial settings. They have now survived two centuries of contact, marginalization, and periods of violence. They occupy a distinctive niche vis-à-vis their respective states and exist as simultaneously acculturated, syncretic, and independent cultural groups. Their economies and their spiritual and material priorities reflect these histories of interaction, which means they no longer fit into Service's typology of tribes.[17] And their self-definitions and self-determining acts are part of their identity as natives. It is the tension of these metamorphoses and the native identities that they produce that have retained my admiration and are so instructive for twenty-first-century global community building.

COMMITTING TO COMMUNAL RIGHTS OF INDIGENOUS PEOPLES

The dual question for this project has been this: What are the keys to communal life, and how committed are we to allowing Indigenous peoples the space and resources to pursue that life? Such respect will allow for cultural self-determination and change but cannot devolve into what Castellino and Gilbert described as the "fear of a continuously available process whereby groups within groups constantly seek to renegotiate their identity and their rights, until being finally satisfied with their bargaining position vis-a-vis other groups" (2003, 164). In other words, if sovereign rights to self-determination are granted to all "peoples," then what criteria or definition establishes a "people" (i.e., having collective rights) from a "minority" or other subgrouping? This is a worry to the international legal community but should also be a subject for literary, moral, and anthropological understanding.

While the ideological and cultural limits on self-determination are set at a simultaneous respect for individual human and collective rights, material limits on this priority for self-determination are set by Indigenous peoples at the capacity necessary given local circumstances. Pursuit of self-determination will also consider appropriate action when communal and individual rights are (or appear to be) in direct conflict. I return to this question throughout the book, but because my own research has been among Native American and Australian Aboriginal Peoples, I rely on the works of other scholars and activists to discuss and test these ideas in a broader (non-CANZUS) global context.[18] Giving more overt attention to the balance of individual and communal processes is, I believe, an important part of the decolonization of Indigeneity (de Oliveira 2009). Further, such a perspective will be valuable to anyone who recognizes the twin and synergistic values of individualism and communalism in every human society.

My own understandings of rights to self-determination were seeded during the Native Title period in Australia in which my research began (see the preface). I first visited the Peak Hill Wiradjuri as an undergraduate student in 1983, immediately after the passage of the locally unpopular New South Wales Aboriginal Land Rights Act. Literally weeks before the 1982 Aboriginal Land Rights Act, the Wiradjuri had agreed to form a Regional Aboriginal Land Council. Only later after the national Native Title Act of 1993 was established did the Peak Hill Wiradjuri put together their claim for the Dumps. It was then that I was invited back to assist in the information gathering. My reentry into that world as an anthropologist (rather than a traveling student) and into the profession of anthropology generally was in the extremely privileged position of having been invited. The strange role of an outsider "helping" insiders translate and perform their culture for powerful others (i.e., the courts) demands acknowledgment. The task for Peak Hill community leaders, and for my mentor-professor Gaynor Macdonald who assisted them, was daunting. Gaynor wrote,

> I'd known Peak Hill people for years, attending meetings and "socials," sharing cups of tea. I knew these claimants were widely recognised as the legitimate "way back" people of that area. The difficulty I foresaw was the absence of written records. . . . And what constituted "credible evidence"? No one knew. Ours was one of the first native title anthropological reports to be prepared in Australia—there were no models, no precedents, and we were working in a state [New South Wales] with the longest history of colonisation. . . . And the fact that this is their country and always has been—which no one contests except white people who've never been to Peak Hill and know nothing about them: "Not our country? Try telling that to my Dad!" An older woman anticipating the court case asked, "What do they want me to do—turn up in some little lap-lap? I know who I am and just let 'em tell me different." (Macdonald 2002, 88)

The intentionality of any Native Title claim and the performed subjectivity mandated in the law itself are modern constructs that anthropologists both embrace and abhor (see also Hart 2018). How the community performed itself for that context and how it gave evidence of its "traditions" would be evaluated by a Western settler nation's court. By definition, an Australian Native Title claim demands that a community be defined and bounded in a way that a court (judge, jurists, a public) can understand. As is the case in many nations where *any* Indigenous rights are recognized, acceptable forms of evidence are outlined in the Australian Native Title Act itself, which calls for plaintiffs to present documentation of their heritage including "traditional" laws and customs connecting them specifically to the land or waters in question. Furthermore, this evidence must be shown to have been transmitted intergenerationally in an unbroken line (Sutton 2004).

Determining how to be a community, how to define oneself as a community to others, and how to engage together as a community in the contemporary era are political and psychological enactments. They are increasingly common performative obligations for Indigenous peoples around the world, as their physical, locational, and spiritual rights are challenged by contemporary forms of encroachment. Not just a logistical responsibility but also a moral project, the tactics and mechanics of Indigenous communalism make up a significant aspect of the cultural diversity we still enjoy in the global context. If we cannot see and witness these mechanisms, how can we hope to preserve or promote such diversity? In an era when economic and ideational forms transgress nation-state boundaries, community building and self-determination will require the same agility and access.

I have worked among many people with a very strong sense of their community: Akimel O'odham Indians living on an isolated reservation in the middle of the Sonoran Desert, Mexican migrants so new to the United States that they have no English skills and a look of constant worry in their eyes, and Australian Aboriginal people struggling through family and grassroot gatherings to piece together their first-ever Native Title claim for ancestral lands. Their sense of themselves as a people was unambiguous, and not just in our conversations about their lives, health, and experiences. It was written into their expressions, their turns of phrase, the way they related to each other and to me. For my part, community was the basis for my interactions with these groups, my reason for being in their lives. So as an anthropologist it has been my assignment to pay witness to their communalism and to recognize it as a relational engagement, not the categorical type into which generalizations so easily slip.

Communalism speaks to the "capacity to culture [that is] a general human right" (Muehlebach 2003). My work gives evidentiary credibility to the claim that assimilation into individualist and priorities is not total, necessary, or acceptable to (former and currently autonomous) Indigenous, sovereign peoples. Indeed, dominant cultures in the world today are not as sophisticated as Indigenous ones in the art and economics of communalism. Their social ties are weaker (see Putnam 2000). They are more dependent on highly technological apparatuses to achieve cohesion (see, e.g., Coffey and Tsosie 2001). And they are often so large in scale as to achieve communalist aspects only through policing and law (Moser 2004). But there are many approaches to peopledom, and if we are serious about communal rights, then both physical (territorial) and conceptual space must be created for this purpose. This is the space needed for communalism.

I have cited generously throughout this text with the intention of giving credit for the legacy of thought informing my own as well as to provide ample suggested readings on the many areas I do not adequately cover. I am sensitive to the limits of one representation, a non-native one, of communal survivance among one Indigenous people. I have relied particularly on others' study of representation, both of and by American Indian / Native American / Indigenous studies scholars. Renya Ramirez captures the creative and resilient work of survivors of San Francisco's colonial past (2007). So too does Martinez Novo, in writing about the strategic identity manipulations by and of, for and against, the Mixtec in Mexico (2006). Although my perspective is clearly an outsider's and an anthropologically academic one, I read the survival of culture and identity despite such barriers as testimony to the centrality of community to shared applied and academic pursuits. This priority, as much as stewardship of sacred and ancestral lands and of political sovereignty, justifies recognition and protection.

Belonging

Generation

Representation

Hybridity

Figure 3. Four features of communalism

Outline of the Book

Using Gila River and others' case data, I discuss four persistent features or processes of communalism. Chapter 1 addresses the first and most personal mechanism, the creation of a sense of **belonging** among members of a community. Belonging is the fundamental sensation of being part of the group, sharing traits or beliefs or customs or goals with others. Of all the traits ascribed to "culture" over the decades by anthropologists, the characteristic of it being *shared* is perhaps the most necessary. Whatever else a community may be, it is shared among the people who belong to that community, and that sensation must be felt individually by each member of the group. There is no culture of one. As members feel some sense of connection to their group, that is, some palpable *communitas*, it is expressed not only in high rituals but in everyday expressions and touchstones. Chapter 1 is an exploration of these communal touchstones.

Second, to build community also requires some self-generating or self-perpetuating element. Whether through the passing on of a community's elements through generations within a family or through ongoing enculturation of new members by those who already belong, the community must sustain itself over time. **Generation** of the community must be ongoing and self-sustained by members in concert with each other. That is, there must be shared patterns into which families and extended groups within the community sustain (or collaboratively revise) those things that give the community meaning and purpose. The concept of "generation" therefore has a double meaning: it refers to the generative process, the creation of members both genetically and symbolically; and it is the intergenerational passage of the community as a whole and to its temporal perpetuation over time. I take up both of these meanings through a grandmother's life in chapter 2.

In chapter 3 I describe how communities must not only tolerate but also facilitate their own meaningful **representation**. This feature of community building relies on the full marketplace of ideas shared and debated across a community. And while there is inevitable conflict, disagreement, and ineffectiveness involved in the representation of any group, a community that cannot be signified cannot be taught, understood, or recognized either by outsiders or by insiders. It therefore cannot regenerate or protect itself. In chapter 3 I discuss multiple meanings and forms of representation, from elected leaders to representational marks on the body. Representation calls upon members of communities to embrace signification and to maximize its useful effects. These various representational projects are typically symbolic processes enacted on a cultural and political stage where the more powerful actors establish and control most representational narratives. But the process of representation cannot be entirely co-opted by the powerful; it is a system of meaning within reach of all members of the group and to outsiders. For native peoples, representation must also be recognized as a historical product. I consider these many representational events through three case studies.

The fourth and final process in community building is, I believe, the most neglected one despite powerful social scientific arguments for its recognition. It is even disparaged in contemporary Western juro-capitalist settings, though it remains absolutely essential and fixed. Fourth is the **hybridity** of persons to be both individualistic and communalistic in culturally distinctive ways. This final requirement of communalism, taken up in chapter 4, requires a recognition of the capacity for change, decision making, and adaptation by both individuals and communities. Recognizing that, in every community, members hold a desire to excel *as* a valued member, the capacity for hybridity between individualism and communalism allows us to imagine alternatives and to reason, feel, and relationally explore change. Hybridity, a fundamental capacity dealt with in fields from behavioral ecology to evolutionary psychology, has a particular valence among social scientists like Homi Bhabha, Marilyn Strathern, and others. For my conversation, hybridity is the quality that allows each individual to invest in the whole in ways that make sense personally. Herein lies the process by which group norms and goals are internalized at the individual level, by which commitment to the group becomes an individualistic pursuit, and through which communal systems might seek and find moral continuity into the future. To assure readers that I am making not a racialized or ontological argument about Indigenous communities but an argument about a universal capacity expressed in unique ways by Indigenous groups, in chapter 4 I draw together behavioral ecology, cognitive anthropology, and psychology and theories of social capital to consider this hybrid communalist agenda. The presence of hybridity is expressed differently across cultures, but the need for internal, individual values that balance selfish and group motives is a requisite element for any community's formation.

After chapters dedicated to each of these four points is a discussion of the ways that community builders have worked to resist and reshape dominating structures of hegemonic individualism in poignant ways (chapter 5). Without straying too far into polemics, this chapter reveals how several Western commercial-legal constructs have stripped away important human, and humanitarian aspects of global relations. In my conclusion (chapter 6) is an argument for the merits of engaged attention to communalism and for global structures that facilitate it. The theory and framing of Indigenous communalism as an intergenerational, relational commitment will be increasingly important for mobile, displaced, and multicultural communities of the twenty-first century. As we ponder the meaning of community for the globalized era, we wrestle with ideas of nativity, tradition, and belonging as communalist forms; with indigeneity and representation as multivalent expressions and experiences; and with the balancing of values determined by all Indigenous persons, themselves dependent on the space in which to deliberate those lifelong choices.

The presence of both communalist and individualist values within each community member creates not a cultural type (e.g., collectivist or individualist) but a basic human capacity. Each of four elements of communalism—belonging, generation, representation, and hybridity—has received its own attention in scholarship since the early twentieth century. But as the arcane typologies of culture have given way to new and shifting forms of community dominant in the globalized twenty-first century, the communal has not been adequately described or theorized. To produce a theory of communal/individual hybridity, whether for academic interest or for applied and policy agendas, we will have to grapple with belonging, cultural generation, representation and its management, and the capacity of humans to blend both individualist and communalist values throughout their lives and over the life of a cultural community. This has been the unique achievement of Indigenous peoples surviving the global colonial forces of the past five centuries, and their lessons are worth learning.

CHAPTER 1

============

Belonging

Living and working within native communities, particularly in the unique space of a reservation setting, often brings with it a heavy sense of community. In everything from daily meals and tasks to large community gatherings, there seems to be more people around by whom one is known and to whom one is obligated. So to help keep peace and harmony in this atmosphere, emphasis is placed on cooperation while individual assertiveness and superiority are limited. Put simply, when you are more aware of the people around you, and they are aware of you, a greater expectation for sharing and fairness emerges. If you have a car, it becomes a taxi; if you have money, you either share it or are a deeply insensitive person to the lack around you; and if you have a funny story to tell, in a place like the reservation, you know you'll always have people that want to hear it.

These are some of the first impressions of difference a Western, individualist observer might notice about native communities. The myriad quotidian ways that all community members add daily to the group's peaceful coexistence are not accidental. High rituals are the more ostentatious symbols and events that denote broadly shared core values and marks of membership; but the everyday rituals and habits of practice, behavior, and thought serve to enculturate members into the group. Indeed, without everyday ways in which core values are learned and practiced, high rituals will become meaningless or hollow.[1]

It is this quotidian element that makes communalism of endless interest to social scientists. Whether examining network bonds, altruistic behaviors, or larger questions of intergenerational cultural patterns, we have long studied individuals' willingness to submit to community restraints. By focusing on Indigenous communalism, I emphasize how Indigenous peoples take a universal human capacity and use it to build relational bonds that span generations and now, in the postcolonial era, form a unique category of peoples. I outline four processes of communalism that are universally accessible by humans, but clarify how, for each one, Indigenous peoples enact their communalist and individualist values in unique ways. And while the intergenerational links connecting Indigenous people to their heritage by blood are part of the equation, autonomous engagements—such as choice, effort, and commitment—also play their role in each of the four processes.

In this chapter, the first of four describing key elements in Pima communalism, I consider three everyday rituals that serve as community touchstones or reminders. These are acts that have struck me as evocative of community yet almost nonchalant in their repetition. I have camouflaged the identities of persons as well as confidential information but have retained the structural elements and patterned speech to reveal how Pimas come to feel, and maintain, a sense of belonging in their unique, internally sovereign community.[2] To achieve a sense of belonging, Indigenous community members do far more than meet constitutional membership criteria. They both are born into a group and place and continuously assert this belonging. The blend of the everyday with more ritualized acts, of singular lives within an intergenerational community, will become clear.

Introductions

The first and one of the most regular aspects of fieldwork in Indian Country is attending meetings of the Tribal Council, so to begin where I myself began, I relate something of those gatherings. Whether explicitly seeking permission to conduct research or attending simply for the remarkable spectacle and process, Tribal Council meetings are a window into formal tribal relations and symbols, a moderately "high" ritual of community. These events are not awash in colors and smoke; in the contemporary era, they rarely involve either dance or song. These meetings have been drastically transformed over time, as one might imagine. At Gila River, the government offices look like office buildings in neighboring Phoenix. There is beautiful desert landscaping, a parking lot filled with cars, an entryway with metal detectors and uniformed officers, and inside the lobby a receptionist speaking English. The building and furniture, the names of the participants, and the language in which the proceedings occur have all changed since 1934 when the tribe established a constitution-based tribal government under the Indian Reorganization Act. But these outward signals can be misleading. There are both ritualized and hidden features in Tribal Council proceedings that remain quite foreign, decidedly private, and certainly unacculturated.

Take for example one recurrent event within this larger ritual: the moment in which each new speaker is introduced to the council and audience. In this unobtrusive and regular act, the distinctions between community members and non–community members are made clear to all who are present. The information contained in these ritualized introductions is conveyed before any other, indicating its importance as a referent for whatever is to follow. Tribal members will identify themselves by family—grandparents or more distant ancestors— location, and (if possible) clan and the traditional name of their community. Whether they speak in a traditional language or in the language of colonizers further situates their identity and their political and social values. All of these details have "deeper dimensions and reflect strong and spiritual connection to the land and other cultural traditions."[3] Here is a typical example of what one might hear when tribal members from different communities are gathered: "My name is John White Cloud Anderson and I'm an enrolled member of the Ojibwe Nation, born into the Bear Clan. I was born in Minocqua and raised on the Fond du Lac by my father, David the Fire Is Burning Anderson, and my mother Mary Day Anderson." Mr. Anderson introduces himself, positioning his remarks within his family (his given tribal name, translated to English, is "White Cloud"), his nation, and several other markers of identity including his parents' names and tribal affiliation. The structure of his introduction is common across all variety of meetings, both within a single group and across tribal communities. And many times this lineal and geographic placement is followed by a few details about the person's experience and work for the community, such as having filled a leadership role, sought education, and returned to serve the community.[4]

Introductions like these have several material functions for communities of an oral tradition, in which knowledge is contained in one's ability to remember rather than one's ability to call upon written records. The detailed but efficient rehearsal of one's lineage serves to allow broad groups of listeners maximum potential to establish some links to the speaker, in shared knowledge, some shared epistemological reference, or relational ties. These links also index not only political and material history but also relevant contemporary authority, functioning much like Western titles and curricula vitae.

But there is another, sometimes greater symbolic purpose to performing one's tribal introduction—even when this information might be written down and available to the audience. The ritual of calling out one's heritage in this way honors those who came before and demonstrates several things. First and foremost, it embodies a position of deference to persons outside of the room, oftentimes ancestors. Bernstein (1997) has described this as a practice of "identity as strategy" and offers a nondisruptive but culturally distinctive performance that itself can have a material influence on an event (Morgan 2007, 281).

Second, those familiar with identity making among Native Americans recognize the invocation of elders and ancestors as a sacrament indicative of an inward spiritual state. The proceedings surrounding any such performance are, thereby, transformed beyond their mundane and profane state into a process with moral gravity. Tribal members who may not have authority to organize or officiate a particular meeting can, through something as simple and brief as an

introduction, transform that event into something more communal and rever-
ent toward the past and elders.[5]

Finally, introductions that reference one's kin place the speaker geo-
relationally. One's past and present filial relations as well as the residential and
cultural choices made in support of those relations (e.g., Macdonald forthcoming, chap. 1) are profoundly informative about a speaker's Indigenous identity.
Whether prayerful invocations or simply testimonies, these verbal utterances
declare Indigenous truths of relationship and place. Erasure of these linguistic
forms would have corresponding ripples to the content they reference.

Relationships and Being Present

It was in a similar realm of tribal committee meetings, introductions, and language that I was struck by a second community touchstone: the value of relationships in community decision making. In the storyline below, I play the main
character, for it is the story of my first major test in the complex political effort
that non-Indians must pass to work in tribal country. When, as a graduate student, I first started volunteering at the Diabetes Education Center, I worried end-
lessly about the inefficiencies and interruptions I met at every turn. I fretted
over delays in hospital workflows and government workers, over the lack of pro-
fessionalism in people who would not keep appointments with me, and over the
inconvenience of endless referrals, new introductions, and "buck passing" by
government and hospital employees who had authority to approve or reject my
proposal for research.

Mine was a typical *Mil-gan* reaction, especially among those who fail to
respect the quotidian presence of cultural difference: those expecting everything
on the reservation to happen as it does in the fast-paced, commodity-driven,
hyperefficient Fordist marketplace of dominant American society.[6] The hammer
of realization would fall on me in one crucial committee meeting, pounding into
me the moral imprint of Pima relational expectations.

I had been scheduled to begin the crucial process of proposals to Tribal Council committees for permission to conduct research on the reservation. My name
appeared on the agenda right after the presentation of an esteemed, midcareer
research physician whom I knew by reputation, representing a globally influential research group. As I describe in *Diabetes among the Pima*, that physician's
well-funded clinical investigation was rejected by this panel of five Tribal Council members. They did not explain their reasons in much detail, but what they
did say focused largely on the failure of the research group's leader to come in
person that day, or perhaps frequently enough in recent history.

Then came my turn. While my proposal was under consideration, only one
question was asked: "Didn't I see you at the *mul-chu-tha*?" The *mul-chu-tha* is

the annual fair and footrace held in Sacaton, the government seat for the reservation and where I usually stayed on work weekends with Pima friends. It is a celebratory event with traditional round-dance music (*keihina*) as well as the more recent dance music *waila* (chicken scratch). The few Mil-gans who do attend the mul-chu-tha are either close friends or family to Pima Indians or are among the more culturally interested staff who work on the reservation.

So the mul-chu-tha was completely irrelevant to my research proposal on diabetes in pregnant women. And this was certainly not an appropriate time for idle chitchat, although that's what I initially thought this was—a way to fill time since no one else had any questions about the research. But what seemed like a meaningless comment to me proved to be an important cue to his fellow committee members about his favorable outlook on my application (without saying so directly, as this would have been too forceful should others have damning information about me that he did not know) and the reasons for his support. Those reasons, he and other council members would later explain to me, had to do with my presence in the community, my demonstration of relationships and commitment to people within it, and my having shown altruistic intentions in my purpose and manner while on the reservation.

Following several more (agonizing) moments of silence, the chairwoman thumbed through her pages and asked if there was a motion. My questioner moved approval, followed by a second from an elder to his left. And my project was unanimously approved at this committee level (and later at the Tribal Council).

It took several years of committee meeting attendance and a familiarity with the many people referenced in casual ways during Tribal Council decision making to understand this lesson. Only one thing cemented my good standing before the Tribal Council committee that day: that I had been seen by community leaders in social settings on the reservation, working a slower pace and with more personal investment than my role as a student, my title as a hospital volunteer, or any office-oriented exchanges would have produced. The extra step was professional, certainly—anthropologists insist on *participant* observation. But it was also personal. I had ingratiated myself to the Tribal Council members (who were strangers) by having genuine and personal connections with a number of community members (not just council members or hospital employees). Even my small network spoke volumes about my intentions and my methodological approach, though I lacked the higher status and title of the physician whose proposal was rejected. As these and a third case show, in the Gila River Indian Community *little* emphasis is given to official titles and positions, much more paid to how speakers demonstrate community relationships and commitment.

Notably, this standard of being present, of relational obligations, applies to community members as well. From research narratives on a variety of topics, I regularly end up with reflections like the one below, in which strong identity, if not also community membership, is achieved only through being present:

> MIGUEL: See when people first got taken out to [boarding] school, just look-
> ing at it now, I think damn, they were crying out for help back then. Even
> then, if you're taking away somebody when you're eight to twelve years
> old—and then losing what our environment, what our people rely on the
> land so much, our belief system, they're just taken out of it, and taken it
> from them, to Riverside [Indian School] and not being raised in our own
> way and how to survive in our environment. When you don't take your
> kids onto the land, my theory is that we lost all of that. And all of sudden
> you come back, you put them back in, and it's a stressful subject. . . . Well,
> how do they know how to raise them O'odham if they're not here to be
> O'odham. You can't be O'odham in California. You can't be O'odham in
> San Diego. O'odham is being here within this certain district.[7]

Miguel is a Pima who has lived on and off the reservation throughout his life (and I return to him later). He voices a regular concern that if you cannot spend meaningful time (including, in this case, one's youth) with and among other Pima, it's hard to learn how to be O'odham.

BUILDING CONSENSUS

My third community touchstone is a fictionalized version of government proceedings, dramatizing the highly mundane and repeated pattern of communication through which tribes enact a blend of Indigenous and Western cultural
decision making. If you have ever sat through a meeting run under *Robert's Rules
of Order* or listened to your local City Council meeting on the public-access station, you know how uncomfortable and frustrating this dialectical straightjacket
can be. More than the unserviceable yoke of imperialist bureaucracy, *Robert's*
hierarchical set of discursive and decisional rules, its committee meeting format, and even its relationship to a constitutional form of governance attempt to
remake the Tribal Council and traditional forms of decision making into something different. Yet so many native communities have resisted these elements of
acculturation. And it is this experience of resistance that makes Indigenous communalism distinct from the cooperative work of others who have not experienced historic subjugation.

To anyone who has witnessed even the public portions of Tribal Council
meetings, this form of discussion and decision making will be familiar. Through
the use of my interpretive account, I demonstrate how relationship work in the
moments and months leading up to votes at a Tribal Council meeting (and not
the voting itself) is a key objective and purpose behind tribal decision making.
In short, the real work of community bubbles up through elders and council

members at those meetings, where it is re-dressed in the bureaucratic clothing of constitutional governance.

In the narrative below, the speakers are a group of elected government (tribal council) members and invited guests, so the traditionally detailed introductions (described above) are not used.[8] Nevertheless, other more quotidian forms of community reference are apparent. In this simple progression, following *Robert's Rules of Order* (1921), an agenda item from a previous meeting is revisited briefly, then tabled for further consideration in another month's time.[9]

What I emphasize in this brief exchange, however, are years-long relationships and obligations behind these interchanges, and there are personal and relational details that are apparent only to those who know all those named actors and the community they work in.

The chairwoman called the next item on the agenda, a proposal for allocation of funds to develop and house a new recreation center in a part of the reservation distant from any other such center. She called on Mr. Antone to speak.

> MR. ANTONE: Thank you, Madame Chairwoman. We will be having a meeting with Cecil Donahue on Thursday to discuss the plan for this rec center. We have also had a community meeting which had a good turn-out. Uh, Ms. Eveline Francis is really leading the initiative on this and has— uh—helping her, has Mr. Howard and Mr. Jackson and—uh—really is most concerned that the elders get an exercise program specifically for them. As uh, as Mr. Donahue said last week when he addressed the—the group over there at the Health Care Corporation, there is a group, there is support from a group of—from the rehabilitation people at the hospital, to see this program going.

Mr. Antone is the elected representative for District 8, not yet an elder, but a member of an influential family in the district.[10] He regularly visits the elders in his own family that live in this district as well as other key elders at least once per month. These visits occur at the elders' homes, at extended family gatherings (e.g., birthdays, funerals, memorials), at community events (e.g., church dinners, elder group meetings, district business meetings), and most often when he is simply walking around the community (e.g., in the district office, the health clinic, or at the school). Because the community is small (the district is home to approximately seven hundred people), elected leaders are expected to be visible and approachable in the community on a regular basis. Mr. Antone is therefore one of the few people who would be trusted to handle such an issue.

Eveline Francis is one of the best known and respected elder women in the district and is well known not only to the members of this committee but also to members of the Tribal Council. Mr. Antone is careful to name her in his remarks, which indicates a nod of deference and respect to her as "really leading this initiative" but also harnesses her authority in support of his own proposal for funds.

Mr. Howard and Mr. Jackson are two more elders in the district, both of whom are known to the committee members either directly or through their families. Their names are used by speakers to indicate real people, not their authorities or offices. This is a repeated and distinctive rhetorical strategy across numerous observed Tribal Council meetings.

MR. BARNABY: [raising a finger to capture the chairwoman's attention]

CHAIRWOMAN: The Chair recognizes Mr. Barnaby.

MR. BARNABY: Has the proposed location been, uh, established yet? And I would also like to ask, has Mr. Juan from the Cultural Resources office been out there yet to look at the site? Because, uh, last month, there was a question, I believe there was a question about the proposed site being, uh, disputed or—that there was some question about the proposed site.

Mr. Barnaby is an elder from a different district. His question is not only a matter of protecting cultural heritage and meeting one's obligations as an elected official but also a performance of his own elder status and knowledge. Mr. Barnaby motioned to be recognized by the chairwoman, rather than the more informal strategy of speaking when a break in the discussion occurred; he named the authoritative and symbolically potent Cultural Resource Management Program, which lent official and bureaucratic importance to his concern; and he demonstrated knowledge of a specific question about the site [a question that, I learned later, was posed by an elder whose name Mr. Antone is not able to remember in the next passage below].

MR. ANTONE: Yes, the original proposed site abutted, was close to property that Mr.—uh, one of the elders there, uh, one of the community members felt was too close to the old . . . there [referencing a landmark documented in oral histories and archaeological records].

MR. BARNABY: Yes, that's it.

Mr. Antone's response to Mr. Barnaby and his demonstration of knowledge about Mr. Barnaby's question were quick and informed. By speaking calmly and with a nonconfrontational expression, Mr. Barnaby conveyed a general sense of support for Mr. Antone's statement and work. Disapproval might have been expressed in a different, likely less direct way, with equal citations to relevant community members. Instead, Mr. Barnaby's comments were a way of helping Mr. Antone to demonstrate further specifics of the community-based efforts he was making and to have these documented for the committee.

MR. BARNABY: Yes, that's it.

MR. ANTONE: Yes, we contacted Mr. Juan and he was not able to come to the meeting last week. I, uh, I don't know yet whether he will be in attendance on Thursday. But—uh—yes, that is one of the items that Ms. Francis and her group are looking into.

Mr. Juan is another Tribal Council member who is *not* part of this committee, but serves in the Tribal Historic Preservation Office, which is responsible
for oversight of historic preservation on tribal lands. Mr. Antone might have
referred instead to a member of the Cultural Resource Management Program
here, since that office is deeply involved in cataloguing and protecting tribal heritage and directly implied by the content of the conversation. But Mr. Antone
made a strategic choice in affirming the importance of Mr. Juan's visit to the site
for two reasons: first, his affirmation showed respect for Mr. Barnaby's concern
that Mr. Juan be involved; and second, it acknowledged the importance of tribal
members (over titled nonmembers, many of whom work for the CRMP) in this
question of heritage protection. Mr. Antone later told me that it was a CRMP
archaeologist who was doing all the work of visiting and researching the proposed site, but that he was a tribal employee and "not the best person" to reference in the discussion above.

> CHAIRWOMAN: So you will have another report for us in two weeks on
> whether that issue—uh, that question, has been answered?
> MR. ANTONE: [gives a single nod indicating "yes"]
> CHAIRWOMAN: Okay. Item is tabled until February. The next item on the
> agenda is. . . .

In this passage, Tribal Council members are working to ensure the proper
community members are involved in a decision of great importance. Western
modes of law and record keeping document this depth of investment poorly or
record it not at all. This is because Western modes tend to acknowledge titles
and offices but may not capture local or micro-level relationships in which those
officers should engage. As DeLanda explains, "The legitimization of organization
through the replacement of individualized actors with organizational 'positions,'
powerful but devoid of personalization" creates fundamentally different networks of interaction and authority (2006, 68–93).[11] Although the deep ties and
relationality of the type in this interchange are not entirely unknown in dominant Western culture, they are a *requisite* in tribal (particularly reservation) communities where *persons*, particularly community members and elders, are
valued more than office. Furthermore, a healthy degree of transparency helps
smaller Indigenous communities avoid abuses of communal authority, whereas
in larger state societies anonymity destroys much of this transparency. Therefore, my provision of details about the many referenced relationships helps clarify what work these actors are doing to ensure, promote, and document a
communal process. Only a person immersed in and knowledgeable about
those relationships would succeed at the level of relational consensus required by
tribal decision making.

The consensus process dramatized in this narrative is one that has been documented in many tribes during and since the period of colonialism (Fry 1976;

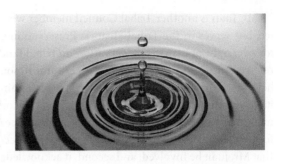

Figure 4. Consensus
decision making extends
through a community like
ripples of water

Johansen 1996; Sutton 2009). I find it noteworthy that this cultural feature can withstand the adoption of other decision-making formats (e.g., republican representation, democratic voting forms) around it. Its importance becomes apparent only when one knows the decision makers, sits through dozens of committee and council meetings to hear their arguments, and spends time with them outside of formal meetings (in the community) where the extended ripples of consensus decision making can be seen. Tribal Council proceedings help create *communitas* by repeating and giving public authority to communal priorities.[12] This process meets the first requirement of community building, to cultivate a sense of belonging and of shared purpose and history.

An Introduction to Communalism

The creation of any sense of unity among a population of potentially disharmonious settlers almost always requires the deliberate agency of man.
—Simon Winchester, *The Men Who United the States*

This work was strictly voluntary, but any animal who absented himself from it would have his rations reduced by half.
—George Orwell, *Animal Farm*

Social and behavioral scientists have long studied the *communitas*, the sense of belonging, among various groups. We have long known communalism to be an important part of any societal project, though there may be a tendency to exaggerate these values in patriotic and nationalist histories. In other words, the giving of priority to the group or the requiring of individuals to demonstrate allegiance to and support of that group, though necessary, has generally been viewed as antagonistic to the individual. That is certainly the case in the United States and many Western political-legal climates. But as Rousseau famously surmised, the alternative to group life is far worse than the sufferings one might endure within a group. "Primitive" man, if left to the limits of his individual resources, would perish and his race along with him (Rousseau [1762] 1978, 52).

However, if primitive man were smart enough to gather "a sum of forces," the aggregation of a cooperating and uniformly motivated group, he could survive. And indeed, this is how we arrived in Rousseau's enlightened epoch: by the decision or accident of human ancestors to live in social groups. Man need only form a type of association (and this is Rousseau's social contract) that engages each individual in such a way that he feels "as free as before," obeying only himself through voluntary submission (though that submission is complete) to no one in particular, but to the whole community. "This act of association produces a moral and collective body, composed of as many members as there are voices in the assembly, which receives from this same act its unity, its common *self*, its life, and its will" (53).

The main problem anthropologists find with Rousseau is an evidentiary one: that his isolationist "natural" or "primitive" man does not really appear in the evolutionary record nor in history. All humans, and even many nonhuman primates, are much more socially bonded and cooperative than Rousseau's idea of primitive man would suggest.[13] Nevertheless, Rousseau pointed us toward the forces of give-and-take in human communal engagement. When societies abridge the rights and freedoms of individuals, they offer in their place some important benefits. Were the collective body not beneficial in such ways, and an appreciable majority of ways we might argue, then we likely wouldn't bother with neighbors, bosses, or even long-term mates.

Anthropologists concur that, whether in the small, kin-based bands of our earliest millennia as a species or in the megacities of modern Mumbai and Beijing, humans generally lead social, cooperative, communal lives. The evolutionary benefits for this coming together in groups have been many: partnership in hunting the megafauna that a single person could never hope to take down; access to a greater variety (and thus greater survival advantage) in mates; shared effort during the seasonal harvesting of large crops for winter consumption or for sale; and collective bargaining power in labor rights or volume discounts at grocery stores. No matter what scale of group, advantages can be wrought from group cohesion, cooperation, and strength.

Thanks to the work of human behavioral ecologists, behavioral economists, and evolutionary psychologists, we can now demonstrate that humans will regularly forgo individual benefits in favor of their membership in a group. We can also show how such sacrifices often convey adaptive advantage to *both* individuals and their groups. Take a solitary cave dweller. She must learn all of the world's dangers by herself. But life in a group gives her constant access to models, both successful and failed, so that she can learn from others' mistakes and thereby avoid them, living a longer or better life as a result. Figuring out who are the most successful, most skilled members of society, then modeling their behavior, is (in behavioral-ecological terms) more efficient. Learners can read cues from those around them as to who has the greatest skill, success, and

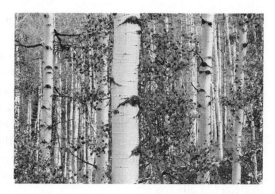

Figure 5. What we see as an
Aspen tree is actually a branch
(or "clone shoot" or "suckers")
off a single root system that
can spread over a hundred
feet from the parent tree.

prestige; or, in the absence of this knowledge, learners may simply copy, or conform to, the majority. Either way, individual success is made much greater by an
awareness of and ability to learn from the successes of others. This is model-
based cultural learning and is something that both is taught to us and is a
psycho-perceptive capacity handed down genetically (see, e.g., Henrich 2004;
Henrich and McElreath 2007; Henrich and Henrich 2007).

Studied in literally thousands of people across multiple disciplinary lines,
altruistic behavior defies simple explanation. Beyond simple modeling, there are
additional benefits that accrue to the group member. Not only are there material benefits in cooperation and the safety of numbers, but humans have built-
in psychoemotional rewards for getting along with others. It just feels good to
be altruistic or to participate successfully in years-long cycles of reciprocity. Personality researchers claim the best predictor of altruistic behavior is something
called an Honesty-Humility personality factor: "the tendency to be fair and genuine in dealing with others, in the sense of cooperating with others even when
one might exploit them without suffering retaliation" (Ashton and Lee 2007, 156).
Research on the purported Honesty-Humility factor and other studies of altruism have shown that this behavior varies by cultural context (Anderson, DiTraglia, and Gerlach 2011), that it is more than an inclination to behave in a socially
desirable way (Hilbig et al. 2015), and that altruism typically favors family members over non-genetically-related individuals, regardless of emotional ties
(Curry, Roberts, and Dunbar 2013). Although this does not explain the factor or
how it works, it captures a set of conditions that can be traced and compared
across groups, bringing sociobiologists, evolutionary psychologists, and anthropologists one step closer to each other.

Not only can altruism pay off in the short term, but even when it provides
no immediate or apparent material payoff to the individual, altruistic acts are
tied to pleasure centers in the brain (Aknin et al. 2013). Thus, while a simpli-
fied economic analysis might suggest that individuals will naturally and reliably behave in a self-interested way, there is substantial evidence that being a

successful member of the group is one of the most "self-interested" things we find to do.

There are too many factors in effective (or adaptive) social life to name. The complexity and number of variables in the process of modeling, the time span involved in estimating reciprocal obligations and payoffs, and the existence of ambiguity in reading social cues or figuring out how to copy good models all affect one's likely success. This means there is an interplay of individual success and group success not limited to individual behavioral choices but that involve a shared understanding of cues—in other words, culture. The cultural system of cues itself can become quite elaborate and will include even (individually) maladaptive choices. One of these that we must address is markers of group membership that are costly or that hurt (see chapter 3). The Henriches elaborate on five evolutionary avenues to cooperation, and even explain how "the scale of cooperation in many societies has increased by orders of magnitude in historical time (Diamond 1997), thereby indicating the presence of some non-genetic evolutionary process that has been ratcheting up the scale of cooperation" (Henrich and Henrich 2007, 41).

In short, people copy the strategies (and even the beliefs) of prestigious and successful others, despite the fact that some of those strategies are not fully or directly beneficial. "Social norms can stabilize any costly behavior" (Henrich and Henrich 2007, 206), including painful markers of group membership (e.g., genital cutting, tattoos) and voluntarily placing oneself in harm's way (e.g., military service). Furthermore, individuals need a group from which to draw ideas and models and thus will also act to preserve that population in which their chosen strategies are proven successful. And here is where communalism comes most fully into view. Learners recognize that success has a context and will work to preserve that context insofar as it is the most suitable arena for the behaviors and choices being made. Preserving one's community—valuing the community for community's sake—is an adaptive value.

The Dangers of Communalism

To prepare and serve a Ham Sandwich, a poor pig's life must be sacrificed to serve the majority of the consumers—that is Utilitarianism. To serve an Egg Sandwich, on the other hand, a cheerful hen must dutifully lay an egg every day to serve the majority of the consumers—that is Communitarianism. In utilitarianism, the means is not important, as long as it produces the beneficial result (consequentialism) for the majority, then it is ethically and morally justifiable. It does not matter if you bomb the enemy's innocent women and children, so long as it maims the enemy's capability to retaliate, then your act is defensible for the greater good of your country. In communitarianism, however, individual life and individual contribution to the community are both

important. As long as you continue laying eggs willingly and happily, you con-
tribute to the common good of the community as a dependable and responsible
hen, I mean, individual.
—Danny Castillones Sillada, *Inusara Journal*, October 8, 2016

The sometimes severe costs to living in groups should be acknowledged. If the Akimel O'odham farmers struggling through the droughts of the nineteenth century *recognized* that staying on the reservation would mean a greater risk of poverty and joblessness, why did they stay? Those costs of communalism promoted departure, rejection of the community—in short, individualism and self-preservation. Even before the droughts and colonization, there were costs—in comfort and health—to living in close proximity with others. But the benefits that accrue from shared historical, psychological, or material bonds must, in an economic analysis, outweigh the costs.

The great city centers have been notoriously filthy, infectious places without aggressive public health and public sanitation controls (Diamond 1987). Communal living also adds risks that would not otherwise be present, or not as great, in more isolated circumstances. Infectious diseases travel more quickly and easily between victims who are in frequent contact with each other. Parasites, microbes, and vermin all thrive where human hosts choose to congregate. About 94 percent of people in the United States today are inoculated against the major infectious diseases, which relieves most concerns one might have for getting diphtheria or polio from one's neighbors. But what about that other 6 percent who are either unable or unwilling to be vaccinated or are ignorantly freeloading off the herd immunity achieved by our larger community?

And while the degree to which societies convince more people to be good rule followers and fewer of us to be cheaters, thieves, hermits, or other rule breakers is a strong predictor of that society's success, there are substantial risks involved if too much authority is given to communal leaders. Communalism for the sake of community can unleash prejudicial violence or other human rights abuses. For example, communal violence in India has erupted in "ethnic earthquakes" as when Muslims are "seen as violent and a danger to Hindu women" (Sengupta 2005). What's worse, Singh argues that the majoritarian Hindu bias has become institutionalized in the agencies of the state (e.g., police, investigative agencies, the judiciary) (Singh 2015). The majority, under a banner of nationalism, thus undergirds majoritarian and religious violence for political ends, turning majority communalism (by nature, not dangerous) into violent majoritarian nationalism. Social scientists have recognized the less obvious but still negative potential of social capital as the power of group connections to do things that are harmful to individuals, the group itself, or externalities. For example, social capital is the set of social resources that holds violent gangs together (e.g., Sandberg 2008). It also refers to the ability of a community to come together as a destructive force or to convince each other to do things that are maladaptive (like smoking or gaining weight together). Or there may simply be an exceptionally costly or difficult communal requirement for membership, as in female genital cutting.

So while group living competes for distinction as one of our most important adaptations, communalism has its costs. For the Akimel O'odham, refusal to leave the community when drought and upstream water theft began to have their effects was a positive force for the community per se, but they then faced several decades of abject poverty living in an area nearly unfit to support human life. In the case of Indigenous peoples worldwide, even the cruel option of abandoning one's heritage and community is sometimes unavailable. Numerous Indigenous groups have been forcibly restricted to reserved lands of frequently poor quality and inadequate size for subsistence. Structural prejudice, societal racism, and legal vulnerability contribute to the distinctive subjugation of native peoples staying put within their local groups for what meager protection they may offer. But individuals also make critical choices, which may vary over a lifetime, about whether and how to invest in their communities.[14] Communalism in these circumstances is a costly moral orientation toward relations and shared history in a communal place, despite sometimes brutal costs.

The Touchstones of Belonging

Santaneros *describe themselves as members of their community by fate of birth. However, community is more than a birthplace or birthright, and to remain an active participant in the social life of the community demands participation in locally sanctioned and defined relationships.*
—Jeffrey H. Cohen, *Cooperation and Community*

One of us, thought Gamache. Three short words, but potent. They more than anything had launched a thousand ships, a thousand attacks. One of us. A circle drawn. And closed. A boundary marked. Those inside and those not.
—Louise Penny, *The Brutal Telling*

Having pondered briefly the larger, evolutionary picture of communalism, I now return to the everyday moments in which individuals come to both feel and enact their belonging in community. Communalist touchstones are everyday events or interactions in which the interests of the community are made evident, and about which individuals' behavior or choices might be judged vis-à-vis their commitment to those interests. I emphasize the everyday touchstones in order to stress the point that communities are built not through monuments and high rituals but through regular, quotidian commitment. Although communities would certainly react if a major ritual were canceled or performed incorrectly, the reaction will be minor over some failure of quotidian ritual. But the persistent and unassuming details reveal themselves over time to have an irrevocable, moral undergirding. In another place and community, these touchstones might involve participation in a Fourth of July parade, attending a certain church or synagogue, or having one's name listed as a sponsor for certain charity events. Communal touchstones require merely some symbol of an individual's commitment to the group, reminding both that person and witnesses what the group's members stand for.

At Gila River, the relational obligations of communalism remain strong. Someone unfamiliar with Native American reservation communities might assume every Tribal Council scenario to be communalist in the ways I've described. But contemporary Native American decision-making practices vary tremendously, blending their long-held community-centered practices with new ones, like Western-style bureaucracy and hierarchy, in myriad ways. In the Gila River touchstones I recorded, council members worked *through* the rules of speaker turn taking, speaker recognition, official votes, and tabling, to ensure long-held traditions are maintained. And it is to these blended strategies that I draw attention.

In innumerable ways around the world, Indigenous leaders resist external forms of representation and decision making in subaltern and creative ways (Scott 1985; Conklin and Graham 1995; Bhabha 1994). They shift the discourse and language of politics. They steer new paths using partnerships with academics, environmentalists, and others who prove helpful (Conklin and Graham 1995; Jackson and Warren 2005; Schwartzman and Zimmerman 2005). The simple act of a speaker's introduction becomes an opportunity to invoke ancestral and place-based forms of authority and rights. What look like Western forms of parliamentary process become weighted with value-laden conversations, delays, and turn taking. Communalism is evident in the tribe's endless work to obtain their rightful water allotments and to care for ancestral and newer irrigation ditches. I also recognized community centeredness in the melodic and influential monologues of elders who bemoaned the declining use of their O'odham language in reservation households or praised the survival of millennia-long farming traditions against stiff odds. And the rewards, in overt expressions and in the visible pride of leaders, were many for the attendance in traditional ribbon shirts of community members needing help with youth programs or the annual mul-chu-tha.

Meanwhile, out in the community and neighborhoods, council members perform consensus work and community by consulting community members in their homes, listening for gossip, hearsay, and other vague but discernible community impressions, and navigating differences and quarrels. They observe and listen in community sites how certain issues, events, or people impacted their surroundings. Consultation with highly connected people directly for their impressions or opinions also occurs, as well as sometimes formal surveying or data gathering. All of these data points are then blended to inform an ideal member's vote on a given subject in the formal meetings of the council.

::::::::::

Our ancestors learned that it is good to take time to meditate, to know what you want and where you are going. Only then should you do it [make decisions] very slowly.
—Anna Moore Shaw, *A Pima Past*

From this perspective, it is easy to understand why, increasingly, non-Indian consultants to Indian Country are criticized for talking too much, not listening, and growing accustomed to strategies that sound like "we'll tell you our plan, and you tell us what you think" rather than "what is your goal for this place, this community?" which is a slower, "nonaggressive" approach and far more likely to promote community over individual offices, titles, or authorities.

In short, the surviving art of consensus building at Gila River both reflects and performs a sense of belonging in the community.[15] There are cultural and traditional relations among the group members: relations of place, of family, of more distant kinship, and of ethnicity that imbue a named leader with webs of obligation.[16] Introductions of the kind I've described above are rehearsals and reenactments of relational webs in these family and place-based webs. A similar system of relational knowledge exists among the Wiradjuri, where "shared history is a highly valued form of Wiradjuri knowledge. Belonging is not based on achievements or abilities. Rather, it requires participation in events and relationships over time" (Macdonald 2004, 22).

And it is important to remember that Tribal Council members can do their job poorly, can succumb to selfish motives, or can simply be fatigued by the work (see chapter 3). Furthermore, consensus decision making can be manipulated or can fail, like any other process of decision making. "There are important relations of power (e.g., of gender and caste) at work in the 'community construction of community,' and an often concealed politics of 'consensus' rule-making. The ability to shape rules and control new institutions, and the ability to use these to 'officialize' private or group needs or social ambitions as the village public good is itself an expression of dominance" (Mosse 1999, 332).

So while tribal consensus building is evidence of a healthy practice of belonging, one need not essentialize these practices. Consensus is a form of managing power and negotiating social exchanges, like any other. Scholars of community certainly recognize that norms of social participation, cooperation, and reciprocity can "become structures for rationalizing social action . . . [such] that their social status is determined largely by that participation" (Cohen 1999, 3).[17]

Key to consensus is that more of the negotiation, information sharing, and statements of position is done publicly and in spaces vulnerable to the subjective and less predictable influence of multiply-intersected decision makers (Andranovich 1995; Steelman et al. 2013). Decisions are not made through secret or anonymous votes. Participants in the process engage with information and other members of the group, allowing more data to reach a greater number of decision makers and for them to be influenced in more transparent ways. And consensus "doesn't mean that everyone agrees about an issue" (Macdonald 2004, 46). It simply means that those present agree to move forward in a particular way. It is about cooperation, acceptance, and trust that the relationships bonding the group together will ensure that everyone's needs and concerns will be addressed over the long run.

Conclusion—More Than Membership

Belonging is the emotional and symbolic feedback that first recognizes members of a group and then reinforces their commitment, but it is not accessible to all Indigenous people. The estimated 370 million Indigenous people in the world belong to five thousand different groups in ninety countries. In the United States, there are 573 federally recognized tribes and over 200 unrecognized tribes. Beyond these limits, Indigenous peoples themselves have rules for recognizing membership, and these vary somewhat around the world.

In the United States, where tribes have the right to define membership, those rules address either blood quantum requirements or lineal descendancy. Whether highly inclusive, like the Sault Ste. Marie Tribe of Chippewa Indians who recognize all descendants of members named on original tribal roles or adopted members, or more restrictive, like the Grand Traverse Band of Ottawas who require one-quarter Grand Traverse Band or Chippewa blood (Fletcher 2012), tribes face increasing scrutiny over these rules.[18] Critics of collective rights argue that both the membership rules themselves and the "privileges" that accrue to recognized members conflict with individual human rights. They argue that Indigenous peoples' rights are already adequately addressed in covenants and laws directed at protections for minority ethnic groups.[19]

It is both an individual and collective right to establish, enact, nourish, and display a sense of belonging within a community. These enactments of belonging vary as widely as the communities to which they are attached. And Indigenous peoples, like all peoples, are flexible in the ways they attach and belong to their community over a lifetime. I have emphasized the existence of cultural syncretism in the form of Indigenous introductions, in the daily commitments to relationships and being present made by Indigenous people, and in the survival of consensus decision making. And while these are good examples of syncretism, adaptation, and survival, these windows onto belonging are not rose colored. I have acknowledged significant risks and dangers of communalism including its potential for obfuscation, corruption, and even violence. There will be inequities of belonging for any people. As Indigenous groups determine the most appropriate membership rules, forms of inclusion and adoption, and strategies for their own communal action and sovereignty, they necessarily balance those communal priorities with individual human rights.

Every community must have its touchstones of belonging—the standards by which members are judged for the genuineness of their commitment and the depth of their sincerity. Not all touchstones are about community reference and loyalty, but the examples in this chapter—introductions, relationships and being present, and building consensus in Native American communities—are deeply communalistic ones. And these offer the first clue as to what is distinctive in Indigenous priorities and values. This chapter has also made a first pass over some of the ways Gila River and Native American communities bond their members together: the touchstones through which the community's values become apparent to and demand certain actions from its members. As I make clear in the next chapter, this cohesion depends on *both* communalist and individualist actions.

::::::::::::

CHAPTER 2

Generation

Transmission [of culture] is a process that may be intentional or uninten-
tional, co-operative or non-co-operative. . . . The recipient of an act of
transmission becomes a transmitter in turn, and the next recipient also,
and so on.
—Dan Sperber, *Explaining Culture*

Everyone needs to have access both to grandparents and grandchildren in
order to be a full human being.
—Margaret Mead, *Blackberry Winter*

Dorothy's queen-size bed, the biggest one in the house, has been the nightly refuge of only two adults over the years. But perhaps a dozen children and grandchildren have taken their turns here, temporary occupants of the relative luxury in space and TV access that grandmother's room affords. The sheets, soft with age, are thin and clinging underneath the ten-pound wool blanket too thick and stiff to tuck or enfold. The mattress compensates for the blanket's refusal by drawing her down into nest-like enclosure.

Dorothy doesn't simply get out of this bed, she has to leverage herself out by swinging her fragile, diabetic feet over the edge, rolling to her side and then push-ing up to a seated position. From there, after a few seconds to clear the fog of sleep from her mind, she drops her head and shifts forward, slowly straighten-ing as if to stack up her bones into the single position that won't produce stab-bing pain.

Lewis, Dorothy's first and only boyfriend and now husband of thirty-four years, is already up and starting to dress. They met and married soon after Dor-othy returned from Sherman boarding school in California. Dorothy loved her high school days and talks dreamily about them as if she were a society debu-tante remembering her years at Hockaday or Choate. Hers was not the experi-ence of her ancestors, shorn of their braids, their language, and their dignity by merciless and militaristic school staff. Dorothy's generation already spoke

English, and she was eager to attend and perform well for teachers and for herself.

Thanks to persistent tribal resistance to the inhumane strategies of assimilation then in place, the 1928 Meriam Report and the 1934 Johnson-O'Malley Act put limits on forced enrollments and cruel tactics within government boarding schools for Indian children. By the 1960s, many reservations had their own, local schools and the government boarding schools had either dropped the inhumane tactics or simply closed. The more recent history of Indian boarding schools is uneven (Stromberg 2006b; Lomawaima 2006) and its impact on a tribes' ability to decolonize education still very much uncertain. But Dorothy remembers boarding school among friends, kind teachers, and a happily busy life that gave her access to better jobs when she came home.

Lewis made no similar trip but was educated on the reservation as a young child and briefly in a non-Indian middle school in a nearby farming town. He has worked on the tribal farm for years, though he always dresses as if he works in an office: ironed denim jeans, a thick leather belt, and a crisp button-down, long-sleeve shirt with all the buttons done. His face and hands are as dark as peppered chocolate, baked to a shiny toughness from years at this job, while underneath his skin is soft and olive-toned. Lewis will be driving equipment in the blazing heat of the fields protected only by his clothing and, if it has one, the tractor cab's roof. For six to eight hours, he'll be out in the desert on the land of his ancestors, coaxing a subsistence out of the desert—though instead of gourds, beans, and melons, he says they're growing crops, like cotton and alfalfa, for sale.

The tribal farm still grows seasonal foods for the community, and we've picked melons together with various grandchildren on a few occasions. But the tribal farm is mechanized now so growing commodity crops helps bring in a larger and more reliable income. The Pima have grown excess crops for sharing, and sometimes for trade, since the early nineteenth century. Lewis is proud to be part of this continuing heritage, and so are his wife and the children. To enjoy such strong ties to the past and to the land gives Lewis a constant source of stability, both emotionally and spiritually, and this purposefulness impacts the rest of the family.

Also like his ancestors, Lewis wears his long hair in one long braid down his back. Now, sitting at his dining table with his first cup of coffee, his hair is still loose and wavy around his shoulders. Dorothy fills his thermos and packs a lunch of sandwiches. They're not talking; the house is quiet and it's dark outside. There are three teenagers sleeping on the sofas just a few feet away, oblivious to this marital constitutional. After Lewis leaves, Dorothy will go back to bed for an hour before she too has to leave for work. This creates a window of opportunity for a grandchild to slip into Lewis's place in the bed.

Such a tiny shift of bodies—making more room in another bed already shared by a mother with perhaps two small children, one of them moving to the privileged space of grandmother's largest room and her company—has meaning within the relationships of waking life. Bed privileges are reserved for adults and the youngest children. So when the house fills up, the older children often make do on the living room sofas and lounge chairs.

And most houses do have children. In 2015, the last census estimates available, children made up 40 percent of the community's population. A small majority of houses (53 percent) are headed by women with no husband or father present. Were Dorothy and Lewis's daughter, Annette, earning the median household income of $30,869 and living on her own with her five children, her home would rank just below the poverty level. But Lewis and Dorothy's multigenerational household is atypical; only 14 percent of Pima houses are multigenerational like theirs.

The fact that Annette lives with her parents is a sign of a current housing crunch on the reservation as well as the lack of employment opportunities (and thus independent income) for those in her generation who do not have a high school diploma or GED. Annette has signed up to receive her own housing from the tribe, but the waiting list is years long. This process is not terribly complicated for applicants, but it does involve filling out several forms with one's home district office and then ensuring that those forms make it through the slow process of reviews. Dorothy, Annette, and several other Pimas complain about the delays associated with bureaucratic paperwork for any task, whether applying for housing, receiving elder benefits, or enrolling for local Women, Infants, and Children (WIC) services. And although I can attest to the slowness of meetings and the likelihood of items being tabled across multiple meetings creating regular backlogs, if not also to the regularity of canceled meetings for lack of quorum, there is good reason for delays. As I saw in so many Tribal Council meetings, the priority is on relationships and consensus building. These take time. One might be criticized for moving slowly, but far better than to move wrongly.

Dorothy's teenage grandchildren are also typical of the 68 percent of Pima kids who are not enrolled in school. Annette did not enjoy Sherman boarding school as her mother did, and she hasn't finished her diploma. Neither did her children's fathers. The persistence of this troublesome school dropout rate is an outgrowth of several factors: the culture clash between communal and Western educational ideals, the limited utility of a high school diploma on the reservation, the bias of social and historical science curricula toward Western cultural content and to the neglect of Native American history and social science, and a parenting model that respects the decision-making capacity of young adults. In this family, completing high school is simply not the norm. So the house remains full and in poverty until someone's income shifts, or their number on the tribal housing list is called.

The family home is itself a symbol of Pima communalism. I know at least a dozen elders who grew up in extended family households, many in houses built by the men of the family. Terri, whom I interviewed in the late 1990s, said her parents had lived in the family "sandwich house"

> until about two years ago, in fact in September. They've lived in the same house my dad built, for thirty-eight years. And then finally one storm came and tore the roof off the house. They determined they couldn't live like that anymore. Red Cross and Environmental Health had to step in and they demolished the house. My dad was standing there watching, saying "I built that with my own two hands. All these years we lived in it, we've added on to it. But now it's gone." He was all broke up, poor thing.

The tribe built her parents a new house since the old one was not fit to live in anymore. And her father wouldn't leave the spot. He insisted the new house be built on the same land. And when they were building it, he hung around to help, to make sure it was built the way he wanted it. Of course the building company tried to usher him away, saying their insurance wouldn't allow him to be on the construction site. But Terri's sister lived next door, so her dad had a permanent and comfortable spot from which to supervise every brick's placement. And he did.

Tribal housing, formerly funded solely by federal sources, is now jointly funded by the community's (nonfederal) funds. Community members can rent government housing or can be awarded housing on the basis of need. Of course one could rent a tiny apartment in neighboring Casa Grande or Chandler, to live surrounded by non-Indians whose values, pastimes, and priorities more closely follow dominant norms. Some Indians do just that. But not in Dorothy's family. The very idea of it is bizarre and unattractive to most of them, and they look forward happily to the day when the tribe gives them their own house. Annette and two other families I knew were on the waiting list in 1999. Within five years all three had received and moved into them (one renovated, two new). The tribal housing office also offers housing repair services to community members, and both Dorothy and Annette had requested repairs periodically. But the wait for these can be long as well, especially for nonessential things like holes in the wall or backed-up plumbing.

The first morning "shift" behind her, Dorothy's second emergence gets her showered and ready for her own job, her tightly permed curls carefully picked and conditioned into a shiny, even mane. Helping Annette or sometimes alone, she'll get the youngest grandchildren dressed, fed, and preened before school, their superhero and Strawberry Shortcake lunch boxes in hand. This too is usually a noiseless morning session, children's needs intimated and met by a multitasking mother or grandmother. Even though the morning is still young and quiet, the Sonoran Desert sun is already yellow and bright by the time this crowd moves toward the car, a Chrysler bought used and on payments when it had forty thousand miles. Three grade-schoolers sit in the back seat, and one joins Dorothy in the passenger seat. Annette drives. No one used to wear seat belts on these short rides, until Annette got into a bad car accident a year ago. Now she buckles and so does Dorothy, even though the car barely gets above fifteen miles per hour on this trip.

They pass ten more cinder-block houses just like theirs, most with a different blanket image darkening the windows—an eagle, running horses, a Bon Jovi album cover in fleece, and occasionally a set of frilled, polyester curtains, drawn back by matching sashes. Every house is silent and dark, the remnants of play and social activities littered around the desert yard—plastic toys and bicycles, mattresses, cars or just their interior seats now serving as lawn furniture, fifty-gallon drums overflowing with debris.

The first stop is the town store two blocks away. If Dorothy gets out of the car, the children will tag along in hopes of begging a soda or snack for themselves as well. If only Annette gets out, Dorothy may give her money and ask for a soda, but not enough for treats for everyone, and the children will simply stay put. They seem to know who has money and when, who is likely to share and who cannot. The day before, Annette had asked Dorothy for money to pay for some clothes for the youngest children, and Dorothy had put her off. Money requests are uncomfortable business in many families. At Gila River, one should be generous and quick to share, especially parents, but children should be responsible and contribute to the family's resources, especially adult children. So there is moral tension involved in money requests, and these can lead to feelings of mistrust and frustration. But the relational work within families includes politics and strategies of sharing. As children learn to balance competing demands and limited resources, they are building moral selves appropriate to Pima culture.

Needs are many in a female-headed family like Annette's. She had struggled for years to finish her GED, keep her WIC paperwork up to date, make the requisite check-ins before receiving her food stamp card, and keep up her family relations (through visiting, sometimes cooking or caring for kin, being present at the many family gatherings). All of this had to occur before she could ask for the help she herself needed. She managed this administrative and caregiving career with an infant and toddlers in tow, unreliable transportation, and the steady requests of others who imagined Annette to be wealthier than she was. Even a high-school-level salary, like Dorothy's or Lewis's, does not stretch very far. And theirs were devoted not only to those present in the household but to family members with lesser claims on that financial source who lived elsewhere on the reservation or even in jail. Carol Stack described a similar circumstance among poor African Americans in the Carolinas, for whom "family life is a resource, sometimes the only readily available resource that poor people can turn to" (1975, 101). So Dorothy was generous in every traditional sense. But Lewis was always a little faster to hand over his cash. Annette knew this and used it to benefit her children and occasionally herself.

Lewis might have stopped at this store too, several hours ago with the truck full of workers carpooling to the farm. They likely bought breakfast tacos from the vendor selling out of the back of a truck in the parking lot. That vendor will be replaced at midday by two more selling fresh *chumuth* tacos: a huge warm tortilla filled with beans and meat. Of course Dorothy and Annette don't buy these—they prefer to make their own. Chumuth are made with white flour and lard like the more familiar Mexican tortillas, but they are thinner and much larger. Annette's nearly cover the two-foot-diameter metal plate she grills them on, and when with the expertise of an artisan she is shaping them into rounds, they expand from a two-inch ball of dough to an even disc draped halfway up her arm. This takes a remarkably short time, only a few seconds, and without the theatrical tosses of an Italian pizzaiolo, producing a much thinner and more fragile textile. After the discs are slightly browned, she folds them twice and stacks them by the dozen, resting a tea towel over them to protect against the ever-present flies. Chumuth is a cheap and delicious form of starch to go with meals of all kinds, but traditionally with beans, chili, and sometimes meat. Another option is *wahmuchtha*, the smaller fried version, also called frybread, for a heavier meal (about 560 calories and eleven grams of fat). These homemade breads are the most important comfort foods Dorothy and Annette can offer their family, despite their obvious role in the local diabetes epidemic. The cooking of these items signals a gathering of the family and brings small but significant contentment to both its makers and its consumers.

With sodas stashed in the moms' purses, the kids are delivered to school, and Dorothy is dropped at the tribal hospital for work, all within a few blocks of the store. Dorothy had recently landed an administrative job at the tribal hospital, a welcome addition to Lewis's respectable salary given their bulging household. Dorothy clocks in with her badge then ambles down several wide, sterile, wheelchair-accessible hallways. The walls are decorated with Edward Curtis photographs, matted and beautifully framed at life-size proportions. Dorothy says hello to certain friends along her route—one at the check-in windows, another at the door to medical records office, another in the nutrition department/cafeteria. She leaves her lunch of a soda and tortilla wrapped in a plastic bag in the communal refrigerator, and tucking her purse into the bottom drawer at her desk, begins a day at the computer screen.

Dorothy's gray cubicle is shaped by the interlocking drawers, file cabinets, and laminate desktops, with the fluorescent lighting coming from underneath the top cabinets. The only visual interruption to this monochrome enclosure comes from Dorothy's family pictures, a postcard from California, and an inspirational poster about teamwork, all secured with magnets from Las Vegas and other bright, colorful destinations. Dorothy is diligent and careful in her data entry, a job that requires a high school diploma, substantial patience with frequently changing protocols and forms, and attention to monotonous detail. She was excited to earn this position, not least because of its pay, its location, and her colleagues. Rarely does she have a complaint because getting a job working for the tribe is a big achievement here, something talked about as a windfall. Government jobs are among the most reliable sources of income one can hope for. Now her family had two of them.

Annette goes back home to nurse the toddlers and vaguely monitor any teenagers who refused to get on the school bus that morning. Later, she will visit her grandmother, Dorothy's mother, in another district of the reservation and take her to church for an afternoon meeting and the evening church service. Dorothy had asked Annette to make the visit to her grandmother's today and help her move a piece of furniture. Dorothy couldn't take the personal leave off work. If Dorothy could get a ride, she would meet them both at the church later. Gila River has several different churches including Baptist, Presbyterian, and Catholic, as well as nondenominational meetings in recreation centers and homes on a regular basis. The fairly strong Christian tradition on the reservation is, of course, a vestige of the influence of Presbyterian missionaries to this area in the nineteenth century. At Gila River, the influence was largely Presbyterian, but other denominations, formats, and even syncretic Christian–Native American church activities now flourish here. Annette has told me, and the greater stability and happiness in her life attest to the fact, that her church community is a profoundly important aspect of her life. Her family members do not all share this enthusiasm, but many will attend services periodically as much for their own spiritual interest as for their interest in accepting Annette's invitations. In this way, Dorothy ensures that Annette's religious life remains compatible with, rather than in conflict with, her family-centered values.

Dorothy's relationship with her daughter illustrates the roles of family and of sharing in this community, and I would estimate among most poor, communal groups. Dorothy also has one son whose coming-of-age experience is also typical of many Pima teens. At nineteen years old, he is in jail for drug-related offenses and will be there the rest of the year. She visits regularly and hopes he'll be released on good behavior before Christmas. Dorothy was initially angry and is frequently sad about these troubles, as most parents would be. But many families have a young member (usually a male, but not always) in jail for several months or more during their late teens or early twenties. Without jobs and uninterested in school, resident youth don't have many legal options for entertainment or income. Dorothy benefitted from the support and genuine understanding of her family and friends, so while her son's legal troubles were a problem, they did not isolate her or create an unbearable stigma.[1]

The jobless youth bulge is a continuous demographic problem on the rez, but it is not a new development. Some incredible interviews were recorded with Pima farmers in 1914, and even these mirror contemporary narratives about joblessness on the reservation. The losses of traditional farming and self-sufficiency, leading to dependence on "the white man" for jobs, water, even survival, have been the fundamental challenge here for almost two hundred years. For example, William Johnson (in the Casa Blanca district of the reservation) narrated,

> We always tried to keep our fences, ditches and farms in good condition. Indians in those days were in close touch with each other. They knew their relation towards each other and cared for one another, but now the white man's laws has [sic] broken up this tribal relationship. Some say it is because there is no water, so there is no use working on our ditches, but I say some are hanging too much on the white man and have little or no respect for their own people. I wish every young Indian boy or girl was like us before the white man came among us. Our fathers have taught us to have respect for our father and mother first and our kinsmen second. So it is today, that some of our young men have dropped and have forgotten their kinsmen and are looking upon the white man as tho he and the Indians were close kin. This is causing trouble, and already some Old Indians have been thrown in jail without good reason. (DeJong 2011, 81)

Culture loss among Pima youth has been bitterly lamented in each subsequent generation, each nostalgic for the past of the generation before. But it is worth noting that many Pima youth from 1914 up to Annette's generation remain on the reservation despite these hardships. In fact for many Pimas, periodic hardships are taken in stride, as Kyle reminded me: "I was supposed to pay for the gas a couple weeks ago and I didn't, and it got shut off. But it didn't bother me. I went back to cooking outside so it didn't bother me." Pimas living on the rez have chosen relations and kin over the potential wealth of advanced education and the possible comforts of city life. In the 2015 census estimates, approximately 5 percent of the U.S. labor force was unemployed, while 32.6 percent of the Pima Indian labor force was unemployed. Behind this striking difference is the fact that 62.7 percent of the U.S. population was in the labor force (that is, either employed or looking for work), while only 47.5 percent of Pima Indians were. In other words, almost 80 percent of the adult Pima population was without employment-based income in 2015. But statistics can't convey what it's like to live in these family-centered ways. The survival of communal living on reservations, despite the regular poverty and need, despite (if not because of) the crowded sofas, beds, and cars, is testimony to a surviving set of values and priorities. Arnold's narrative of hardship and poverty, like Kyle's, is not a dejected and exhausted one; it is a narrative of good times and family memories: "There are a lot of kids in our family, and you've got to make things stretch, eat a lot of beans and fried potatoes, stuff like that. I guess people call it poverty but I didn't see it as poverty. We always had enough to eat. We didn't have all the good things the other kids had, but we made do, we had fun." Dorothy and her family's morning routine is steeled by the pervasive, intergenerational poverty that her community has known since it lost its water to white settlers upstream.

What the poverty statistics belie is not just the absence of income but an intentional rejection, in part if not in whole, of the commodity-fetishizing lifestyle of the dominant settler culture. Commodity fetishism is an idea of Karl Marx that, along with profit-seeking capitalist production, changes the value of things from value related to their utility to value determined by their ability to fetch money. With this transition, we as humans have forgotten that value rests in relations among people as they work to meet needs and comforts; we now think the commodity, the product, has inherent value simply and solely because of its power as a commodity. The value of a brand name captures this idea—that a brand name rocking chair has greater value than an equally well-crafted rocking chair of an unknown brand. Commodity fetishizers seek to purchase not only goods that they need but commodities of a certain status, if you will, often reflected in their price.

But commodity fetishism has not displaced relational values at Gila River or in communalist Indigenous groups. Here one can see a different set of values, such as rejection of an education that orients a person toward a type of success most likely found too far from home and family; rejection of housing that might meet a commercialized standard of status or function but isolates a person away from all the people, places, and daily experiences that make life enjoyable; and rejection of an education that neither includes Native American history nor foments a future within one's heritage. These are decolonized priorities and forms of cultural survival.

Ultimately, within the communally vibrant Gila River and certainly in Dorothy's family, there is also a pattern of noncondemnation for individual errors, rule breaking, even illegal activity, as well as a high tolerance for personal choices of others, even children.[2] Certainly parents (and grandparents) make instructive comments to children about school and responsibilities, but children are given latitude to make mistakes in certain areas of life. Whether because of different values, different culture, or intergenerational change, the individuality of Pimas—even young ones—is recognized and valued. People are held accountable for their actions, and individual achievements and qualities receive their due accolades. But with respect to wealth and some of the material aspects of life, reservation life remains a relational economy in many ways. Families should produce what they need to care for themselves and their community, and wealth accumulation is often seen as greedy, selfish, and not very "Indian."

Generating individuals into this system of priorities is a loving indoctrination. It is a process inherent to all cultural groups everywhere. In family and even public settings at Gila River, I witnessed so many instances of this process that their meaning and import were, for a long time, invisible. Those cultural priorities that are infused into each member's life in unnoticeable ways produce the most stable forms of habitus, especially when those priorities for the group appear to members as if they have chosen their own paths.

INDIVIDUALS IN A COMMUNAL CONTEXT

Freedom (n.): To ask nothing. To expect nothing. To depend on nothing.
—Ayn Rand, *The Fountainhead*

This kind of thinking, he found, is not the way to make oneself popular with other birds.
—Richard Bach, *Jonathan Livingston Seagull*

The term "generation" has multiple meanings. I use it primarily to emphasize the generative work of raising, training, and influencing the values within each community member. By focusing on "generation" rather than "raising" or "encul-turating," I'm calling up the deep investments of kin and kin-like relations within the networks of community members. These influencers are motivated to promote like-mindedness within a family, and while their work may not always be overt or even conscious, the net effect is a stronger, more integrated web of social bonds.

A second reason for using the term "generation" is for its indexical capacity for multiple generations of family and of a community. Clearly this multigen-erational history is especially important to Indigenous peoples identity. Not only are the links between Dorothy, her daughter, and grandchildren relevant to our understanding of how communalism is nurtured, but further links backward and forward in time merit closer attention. For the Pima, as well as for the Wirad-juri and native peoples worldwide, this generative work is about longevity and survival beyond the current living members.

Finally, but in resistance to assumptions about genes and descent, I use the term "generation" to draw attention to affinal and adoptive relations that exist in all communities and certainly within Native American peoples. Inclusion of certain non-Indians within a community is fairly common, though these may or may not be legally recognized for a variety of reasons (Kenrick and Lewis 2004). As I alluded to briefly in the last chapter, tribal membership rules do not accomplish the equally important goal of members having a sense of belonging in the community. This comes only from relational engagement and commit-ment over time. In this chapter, I focus on that accumulation of time and the long game of Indigenous lifeways.

I have already described native communities, including the Pima and the Wiradjuri, as members of what anthropologists call communalist or collectiv-ist societies. Giving greater priority to the group and minimizing individualism are what anthropologists have for more than a century considered hallmark traits of tribal and small-scale societies, of groups around the world whose economic subsistence depends more on cooperation than, for example, groups living indus-trialized lives with wage-labor economies. Over time, a communal society member's character is assessed against these obligations to the larger group.

Thus, the question is raised, what makes a "good" Indian in these communi-ties? Must "good" Indians perpetually think of their people/village/clan/land before themselves and tamp down their selfishness and self-importance in reg-ular ways? In contrast are individualists who prioritize self-preservation and per-sonal gratification, who engage with the social world only insofar as it serves oneself "bad" people? Without overdrawing these distinctions, it is useful to reconsider these two ideas as moral values on a continuum, each one being acces-sible to humans in different contexts. In this chapter on the *generation* of new community members—the raising of Pima Indians to be "good"—the difference between communal and individualist becomes less clear. Individuals *within* community must make daily decisions about what is "good," including that what might be harmful today may achieve a greater good in the future.

To understand the individual within the community, it bears reviewing some of the historical treatments of communalism and individualism in the social sciences. What assumptions might exist about these ideas, about how they are taught and achieved in particular moral worlds? In the broader U.S. culture, we know best what individualism looks like. For example, our society gives indi-viduals the right to choose whether they brush their teeth, drink alcoholic bev-erages, or stick closely to the posted trails in Grand Canyon National Park. As state-size societies grow, they become dependent on institutional platforms like a legal code, a national park service, or a(n inadequate) funding structure for the policing of public behavior. Such institutions give citizens certain rights to choose and to enjoy or suffer the consequences of their actions. Disregarding the fact that two or three deaths occur every year from falls in the Grand Can-yon, typically because someone ignored posted warnings, or because the 1,450-mile Colorado River creates an unfenceable rim perimeter (Ghiglieri and Myers 2001), the individual drive for freedom and personal gratification is a fundamen-tal value undergirding many U.S. societal institutions and cultural norms.

Aspects of Pima individualism are also apparent in the early hours of Doro-thy's typical weekday. Pimas learn how, when, and whether to share money. Small children learn the meaning of school and the value of that education. Teenagers observe and test various forms of freedom, work, sharing, selfishness, isolation, and communalism to suit their circumstances, their personality, and their cul-ture. As teens emerge into adults—sometimes before, oftentimes well after they have had children of their own—they are held accountable for their actions and words vis-à-vis the family and larger community. Achievements are rewarded in family and public ways, while errors and abuses are punished by social or legal sanction according to their severity. In watching these dramas unfold, Pima children learn norms for freedom and jail, schooling and unemployment, sharing and lifestyle. Even in this communalist setting—and a family-centered case study within that communalist setting—one can see the opportunities for more selfish individualism, how it can emerge, be expressed, and even thrive in distinctly Pima ways.

The character of individualism (or as Kusserow would say the "individualisms") within any cultural group is evident in writings of and since the Renaissance. Philosopher Thomas Hobbes, whose ideas on the social contract are both influential and well known, was reflecting on his own society's experience after England's mid-seventeenth-century civil war. Civil and political leaders fired by the promise of new freedoms also had to keep individuals from destroying everything in their search for autonomous authority. John Locke, who dwelled on the natural rights of man regardless of government structure, was influenced by the same political climate. What these well-known Western scholars have in common is a (political) view that individuals sacrifice only some of their rights in exchange for a government of laws; and that individuals did not owe their complete dedication to sovereigns in exchange for the safety and benefits of group life. Individual autonomy may have been fundamental in these new civil societies, but it was still predicated on some degree of submission to communal needs and demands.

Western individualism would take on new elements in the late eighteenth and nineteenth centuries, with the invigorated laboratory of the Enlightenment. Experimental science, global circumnavigation, exploration, and ethnology would together inspire the modern age of political philosophy. Hume and Kant helped shift our gaze downward from the heavens and inward to the bounded individual body. For them, the individual had both life and consciousness of that life. These and other late Enlightenment (1780–1815) philosophers gave character to this individual whose nature was good but whose experience could go afoul of the church and its teachings (e.g., Rousseau, who wrote flatteringly of "natural man" in primitive states, free of the vices of private property in *Discourse on Inequality*; or Kierkegaard, whose individual was in its true form a relation with God and was ruined or distracted by relations with "the public," in *Works of Love*; although see also *Papers and Journals* [1996]). These ideas were not openly hostile to religious doctrine of the time but certainly reflected a society moving beyond its restrictive religious history.

Over time, theoreticians would draw distinctions between government types, recognize the cross-cultural variation in the characteristics of esteemed leaders, and even explain "the state" as both an ethnological subject and a theoretical abstraction (Service 1971). Out of these experiments, the political frame of liberal individualism would take hold—the view that the individual is the original and primary unit of social organization, someone who exists prior to the community (rather than someone formed through it, for example, as we will learn from Mauss and others momentarily) and who is the subject and basis for societal functioning.[3] This frame, and the high value placed on individualism that goes with it, would inspire revolutions and transform governments (e.g., Macpherson and Cunningham1962). Individualism is a value that binds together particular legal, political, and economic institutions in a powerful way, making it difficult to challenge or even question.

WESTERN INDIVIDUALISM

Liberal individualism's hold on our concepts of persons and human rationality and our freedoms of choice seems overwhelming and irreversible. For one thing, the global apparatuses that sustain individualist laws and person-centered rational thoughts are ubiquitous and hegemonic. But even further, for a scholar to question individual autonomy is tantamount to a human rights abuse. So one must step gingerly among the assumptions of this political framework and consider them as constituent parts to a cultural whole.

The essential concern, as I introduced last chapter under the heading "costs of communalism," is the risk of communal tyranny and abuse. But both communitarian ethicists and advocates for Indigenous and collective rights affirm that a number of individual human rights not only tolerate but *require* minimum protection of collective formations. Individual rights to, for example, religious freedom and political participation demand that individuals can exercise autonomous choices. "Autonomy in thought and action is thus seen as necessary for the exercise of other liberal values such as self-respect, happiness, critical reflection, and liberty" (Thompson 1997, 787). To meet this standard, the Universal Declaration of Human Rights (UDHR) affirms our individual rights to "realization of the economic, social, and cultural rights indispensable for his dignity," "to manifest his religion" (Article 18), to "free assembly and association (Article 19), and to "participate in the cultural life of his community" (Article 27). To enjoy their individual human rights, Indigenous people must therefore have access to space (i.e., traditional lands, communities, collective autonomy) on and through which they can practice their heritage, their religious life, and their identity.

To better understand the individual to whom the UDHR rights adhere requires an awareness of Western notions of the individual or personhood and the characteristics assumed to belong to that entity. It is because of this universal capacity and experience of humans—regardless of legal categories differentiating slave from free, male from female, or greater group from lesser group—that universal human rights were declared. Certain rights were determined to adhere to all humans because of that species' intellectual, emotional, and cognitive makeup. These rights do not adhere to other animals or organisms. A first constituent of the Western individual or person deserving rights is, in short, her rationality—her ability to think, consider information, and form judgments by a process of logic. These qualities were considered by Aristotle to be distinctive to humans and reflect assumptions fundamental to the UDHR.[4]

For the Greeks, rationality, which may seem most familiar to readers, required the clear formulation of a problem and the specification of any assumptions— for example, assumed values, priorities, or views on the nature of the world. Once these assumptions and the problem were established, several more rules for rationality applied: (1) it must be based in reality or cause-and-effect relationships; (2) it requires the application of intellect and deductive reasoning to a given problem, as opposed to purely creative or imaginary modes; (3) imagery and creativity are cast out and replaced with regulative and standardizing cognition (Verran 1998); and (4) knowledge must be "non-contradictory" (Young 1981, 318).

A variety of such rules for "rationality" have emerged, across different disciplines, since the classical era. Max Weber outlined four different kinds of rationality (practical, theoretical, formative, and substantive) (Kalberg 1994). In the field of economics (e.g., Hollis and Nell 1975), individuals may be theorized as *perfectly* rational, meaning that they will act in ways that are ultimately useful to them (an assumption that defines utility as that which individuals decide is optimal). And in evolutionary biology, rationality is also surprisingly economic but population driven. Individuals are perfectly capable of poor choices, but only successful individuals contribute to the gene pool. Finally, in contemporary anthropology, rationality may be more socially informed because it recognizes how individual biologies must adapt in social worlds (e.g., Young 1981) and how rationality can and must tolerate paradox and ambiguity (Sykes 2012). Anthropology's cross-cultural perspective lends the advantage of comparison, making both conceptually possible and visible a multiplicity of forms of rationality (or of individualism or communalism). Thus, the ethnological approach recognizes *multiple* ways in which humans can think about causes and effects, the relevance of imagery, or what makes up intellect—the elements of rationality listed above.

Recognizing the cultural variation in rationality, one must concede that the rational individual might, therefore, produce individualist or communalist decisions for different reasons in different contexts. Rationality and individualism are, thereby, decoupled from the ontological coupling given to them in much of Western liberal individualism. By the mid-nineteenth century, scholars had begun to use cross-cultural study to inform this decoupling and to understand both individualism and communalism better on their own terms, the rationalities that sustained them, and the relationship of these values to societal function. Alexis de Tocqueville, a nineteenth-century social philosopher compared European individualism to its American cousin, acknowledged that these differences were, at least in part, attributable to the historical and even environmental features of each location. Others like Kroeber, Kluckhohn, and Mauss seemed to chafe against the ideological assumptions of their own heritage and worked to understand native and colonized communities in more emically correct ways.

Marcel Mauss, social scientist and nephew of Émile Durkheim, deserves special attention here since his was a formative essay for anthropological challenges to individualism. His historical and comparative method revealed personhood as something that had evolved through a succession of forms: "From a simple masquerade to the mask, from a 'role' (*personnage*) to a 'person' (*personne*), to a name, to an individual; from the latter to a being possessing metaphysical and moral value; from a moral consciousness to a sacred being; from the latter to a fundamental form of thought and action—the course is accomplished" (Mauss [1938] 1985, 3). Mauss's origin point for the person was the Etruscan mask society. The Latin etymology for "person" being sounding (*sona*) plus through (*per*) led him to hypothesize that the person's origin lay in these early masked rituals: the person was formed by "sounding through" the mask, or through one's roles in society. Mauss studied one of the earliest Roman rituals as a window onto those prior Etruscan societies. He found clan-like groups were *personae* (individuals), not just the users of masks but the living entity of importance to society. Masks were linked to rituals and privileges within a communal system, such that individuals filled a role in society through their assigned mask, sharing in the life of the larger organism, indeed having their life *through the role that they played*. The mask did not cover a preexisting entity; it was the vehicle to an identity, to full personhood. In other words, full personhood (or full humanness) meant social or communal engagement.

According to Mauss, from this masked individual, human societies made a short conceptual jump to ownership (or inheritance) of heritage, tying individuals to their inheritance group (i.e., lineage) and not to the broad community in which the role took its meaning.[5] This evolution, this progressive conceptual excision of individuals from their original and defining society, made possible the later Roman individual citizen and the Christian individual soul. It would also form the ontological and cultural break that native groups around the world must constantly resist if they are to survive as cultural groups. Indigenous styles of authority are often undermined in organizations that privilege institutionalized roles over the lifelong relational authority of members in relationship to one another (see Macdonald 2018; Brady 2007).

Anthropologists have had nearly eighty years to reflect on Mauss's person-as-role theory. Several are useful in the pages ahead, including Louis Dumont (1980) and his comparison of Indian personhood—viewed to be fundamentally hierarchical and inextricably communal—and American personhood—viewed as fundamentally equality driven and therefore individualistic. By the middle of the twentieth century, this binary conceptualization of individual *versus* society as a way of characterizing cultural groups or societies came under scrutiny. Scholars like Dumont, McKenna, and Strathern took their cues from earlier theorists like Mauss and Geert Hofstede to begin recording the variations and permutations between individualism and communalism present in the world. Others have written ontological, psychological, even metaphysical explorations of individuality as personal experience and human condition (Burridge 1979). These works have been helpful comparisons in my own study of Pima communalism, as is apparent in the pages ahead.

Today, individualism is recognized as highly variable across settings. Individualism is not even an inevitable or homogenous experience in Western culture. Kusserow illustrates this in powerful ethnographic detail in her study of three *types* of American individualism. This value is not only learned but expressed in tremendously different ways: "Individualism has many different strands, meanings, definitions, and forms that are taken up differently by various individuals, local worlds, and subcultures. It is a large enough public symbol to include a multitude of meanings. Its power lies precisely in its ambiguity and plasticity, in the ways different groups can espouse and use its different elements and meanings to fit their local context" (Kusserow 2004, 21).

Kusserow's work helps bridge the span between anthropology and psychology, the latter of which is a field far more interested in the individual perceptions, productions, and self-construals of these values and behaviors. And over time, anthropologists have elaborated multiple forms of the individual and individualism, exploring ethnographically how "individualistic styles" form and vary in differing circumstances and contexts (Carrithers, Collins, and Lukes 1985; Hsu 1983; Kusserow 1999, 2004; La Fontaine 1985). Through this repeated and deep mining for detail, we have affirmed that the individual is acknowledged in some way in all cultures, that its definition and roles are of paramount concern to each society, but that individualism and communalism are better conceived as values upon which all humans draw than as taxonomic categories to differentiate between entire groups of people.

Finally, Western individualism has been a highly gendered expression, having itself emerged through gender-biased writings out of a patriarchal history. I cannot address these biases here, but it is worth noting that the Indigenous women's movement not only has been influential in promoting gender security and justice but also has been pivotal within broader global Indigenous activism (e.g., Sieder and Barrera 2017).

Pima Individualism(s)

As a grandmother cares for her family, Dorothy is teaching its youngest members how to nurture, to be elder, to be female, and to be Indian. Whether and when she shares money, the way she responds to teenagers who skip or drop out of school, how and where she works or spends her free time—all of these and myriad other acts carry lessons about Pima culture and the values of family and community. The generative power of Dorothy's weekday morning routine is one of the fundamental mechanisms of culture and cultural transmission that so many anthropologists have pursued over the decades. But beyond this, these are *active* forms of resistance to Western customs of family making and individualism; the preservation and honor of these forms of *generation* are decolonizing acts (Waziyatawin and Yellow Bird 2012).

Coded into each moment when she may (or chooses not to) make a complaint are a blend of Dorothy's personal values and community norms. In a single morning, I witnessed norms expressed around freedom, jail, employment and unemployment, educational achievement, expressions of family love, parental responsibilities, the value of money, dietary ideals, and cultural foodways, to name just a few. Rather than tease each of these out (one could write a book on each subject), here I witness the work of enculturation that occurs in so many expressions and actions of daily life. The generation of "good" Pimas involves the primary actions of parents and extended family, particularly elders.

Perhaps because of the substantial cultural change that most Native American groups have experienced in the past two centuries, there seems to be a broad tolerance within the Gila River Indian Community for multiple ways of surviving, even thriving, *as* Pima. Pima individualism, like individualisms across cultures, is enacted differently according to one's context and experience. For example, Pima children are expected to be respectful of adults, but when they have periods of rebellion and laziness, they don't lose their identity. The same can be said for living in nuclear family homes rather than extended families or having smaller families or no kids at all. But there are limits to what is recognized as good Pima behavior or living in the Pima way.

One of the strongest markers of Pima identity, either permanently or periodically in one's life, remains life on the reservation. Much has been written about "reservation life," so I do not repeat those lessons here. David Treuer, who wrote an unblinking account of reservation life, says that "life is hard for many on the rez. If the usual story we hear of life on the rez is one of hardship, the subplot is about conflict" (2012). But a good many of the Pimas I know insist that Pima identity is strongly influenced, if not dependent upon, time spent on the reservation. Native Americans protect and preserve their access to these places not just because they're the geographic location of their birth or current residence but because of their connections to family and community going back generations or even millennia. Active and renewable commitment to those common sources of heritage, tradition, and belonging both symbolizes and is a sufficient (although not always necessary) cause of community. I discuss the rez and notions of place more broadly in the final chapter since these have much to do with native identity, transmitted culturally and through families and traditions. For now I focus simply on the generation of new community members and "good" Pimas in a particular place that they have always shared.

The second major characteristic of Pima individualism is its relational ethic and the presence of multiple social networks in every person's life. In the conversations I have quoted, speakers have drawn influence from a "general" social community—friends, family, and unfamiliar community members whose own behaviors or comments impacted them in some way. Macdonald's description of Wiradjuri individualism is similar: "All individuals are expected to realise their personal responsibilities, and thus their social value, by sharing. . . . Being a Wiradjuri person comes about through relationship, not through attaining a role: husband, or mother, or by gaining a qualification such as teacher, carpenter, nurse. A Wiradjuri person *exists in relation* to those with whom they have a sharing relationship" (Macdonald forthcoming).

Included in these formative relations, but particularly powerful and formative to how Pima individualism is achieved and expressed, is the family. Dillan is a young father working as a full-time warehouse clerk and raising his children on the reservation. He was part of a regular Saturday pickup basketball game at a rec center on the reservation, with four or five other twentysomething men. Two in the group were brothers, most had known each other for many years, and occasionally others, including women, would enter the game. On one Saturday I brought some snacks and this group offered to talk with me about life on the reservation, its stresses and joys, and their ideas about Pima tradition and family.

Most of the men in this pickup basketball group had, and lived with, their children. And although they described fairly typical issues with their partners and parenting, they were by most measures successful: most lived with the mother of their children; their children, albeit still mostly young, were attending school and reportedly well-behaved. Dillan said that although he teaches his kids to mind their parents and respect their elders and family, he would expect "anybody who knows what they're talking about and what they're doing" to tell him if his kids were "in trouble." This is an adult's responsibility for any young person, since "in the traditional way, eighteen is not becoming a man. It's when you have to go through a series of trials and obstacles before you can say that you've become a man. When you turn eighteen that's just the law's way of saying that you've become an adult. In our traditional way we don't see eighteen as becoming a man." The other men, about five of them, nodded in assent. Young people do not magically become mature at the age of eighteen. It is an adult's responsibility to help influence Pima children and teens to become "good" adults. (In another conversation, one Pima mother invoked the oft-quoted saying "it takes a village.") Then Kyle, a friend of Dillan's in the group, spoke up to suggest a limit on this communalist pressure: "It depends on if I know them or not. I don't really stick my nose in other people's business. I pretty much stick to my own or my family." Family, then, if not just *any* community member, is reliably expected to advise and intervene if a young person is getting into trouble, whether drinking or drugs, dropping out of school, or simply being disrespectful to elders. The consensus in this group, as they took a break from a pickup game of basketball, was elaborated with jokes about the role of family members in addressing problem behavior, but also rewarding each other with attention and caring. In many instances the ideal family seemed more elusive than real, but all agreed that family, especially in its extended form, is the first and most important referent for Pimas.

This is family centeredness or familism, which has been theorized as a core cultural value for Latino and native peoples in many settings (Guillory and Wolverton 2008; Smith-Morris et al. 2013). A collective form of decision making and responsibility, familism occurs in parallel with the larger communalism at Gila River. It requires the individual to ensure the well-being of family members (both nuclear and extended). And for those judged or believing to adhere to this value, the family is a source of emotional comfort, support, and even health benefits during the stressful periods of unemployment, illness, or family crises and major events. Familism was certainly an apt description of the values expressed by this basketball group but is vibrant among Dorothy and Annette as well.

Now, family can also be a primary source of conflict, shame, or stress for the individuals who subscribe to this value. Familism can be a source of surveillance and pressure, which threaten to shift a person's allegiances and devotions to others.

> FRANCINE: I don't know. Because I don't feel right. My old man used to tell me I was fat, fat bitch and that kind of stuff.
> ARMAND: Oh, and me and my girlfriend had an argument and I ended up getting mad, so I busted out her car window. It's just normal. Sometimes people call it "Indian love."

So clearly family is both a positive and negative force. In my approach to Pima families over the years, I have taken a multi-form and "multi-local" (following Foner 1997, 2003) view of familism. For Pima families, some members move off the reservation while most stay and the proximity of reservation life brings constant shifts and transformations to family balance. I am convinced that all cultures undergo a measure of this type of metamorphic pressure over time, but some groups adhere more closely to familism or to communalism. The boundaries of one's primary reference can be expected to shift somewhat over a lifetime.

In sum, Pima individualism is multifocal but prioritizes community, family, and the shared space of the reservation. Poverty and other hardships are not so devastating as to make people want to leave their community—not now and not in 1914 when recordings were made with Pima farmers about their years of struggle with dry irrigation canals, loss of water to upstream whites, and barely avoiding starvation by selling mesquite wood from the desert (DeJong 2011). "Good" Pimas are generated, as all cultures are generated, through the relational acts of kin and community as they practice the core values, traditions, and ways of being Pima together; not in strict conformity to past or "traditional" ways but in ever-new interpretations and applications of the lessons of those who came before.

GENERATING COMMUNITY OUT OF INDIVIDUALS

When Indigenous right advocate Jeff Corntassel wrote that self-determination is incomplete if it is not sustainable, he was speaking not just to issues of change but to intergenerational change. The capacity for intergenerational transmission of culture (the second meaning for this chapter's title), including ways of being a good Indian, requires attention and resources. Corntassel wrote, "For Indigenous peoples, sustainability is intrinsically linked to the transmission of traditional knowledge and cultural practices to future generations" (2008, 118). This capacity includes and is embedded within "the interlocking and reciprocal responsibilities to one's community family, clans/societies . . . , homelands, and the natural world" (118).

But for many communities, only a "fragmented Indigenous identity" survives in the postcolonial era, during which Western cultural forms of government, education, and economies are constantly pushing at the boundaries of Indigenous communities and identities (Wickham 2012, 181). Native American youth are rising to lead their communities with still-limited resources in decolonized forms of leadership. Natives (and some anthropologists) recognize a broad diversity of patterns in how people modify their cultural value systems, such as familism or communalism, in response to pressures and challenges. They observe and can record mechanisms of *generation* that promote communal values and sustainable living in relation to both each other and the earth. And through self-determination, native activists and scholars are now promoting decolonization and forms of "survivance" (resistance + survival) (Stromberg 2006a; Powell 2002) against domination by non-native ideologies to ensure the continuation of Native American communities in traditionally respectful yet future-oriented ways of living.

In this light, constructs such as communalism and familism offer an explanation of native peoples only as a whole and historically. Such general constructs are less adept at describing the dynamic and malleable ways that individuals think and act vis-à-vis their community throughout a lifetime. Consider the mutability of families within many cultural groups—their boundaries, definitions, and roles—combined with the myriad ways that devotion to this group of kin might be expressed. I have argued before that although familism may be present over different times and circumstances, other terms may be more accurate to describe this orientation toward kin (Smith-Morris et al. 2012). Namely, one's devotion to family and the crafting of one's identity around one's family might be better understood in the broader terms of social interdependence or connectedness (Halgunseth, Ispa, and Rudy 2006). Familism might simply be a particular form of communalism. What these two constructs share in common is actually a type of individualism—a personality of sorts—that defers in certain decisions to one's larger kin or communal network. Both familism and communalism arise in Pima narratives and are central to the generation of "good" Pimas. Yet, in context, neither of these constructs can be effectively described as monolithic or homogeneous in their appearance among Pimas. Likewise, there is no single way of being individualistic. Each of these terms points to a cultural ideal that reveals itself in complex ways. Learning how to be a proper individual is just like learning how to be a proper community member; these are two ways of saying the same thing—being a "good" person in a particular society.[6]

::::::::::

Dorothy and Lewis are typical Pima grandparents. They participate in reservation life and some of the same Pima lifeways that stretch back into history longer than they can remember. But they also made changes and have lived differently than their own parents and grandparents. They drive cars, earn a wage for work on the farm or in an office, eat store-bought foods (some of it bad for them), and struggle with the problems of poverty, crime, and unemployment that impact so many living on the reservation. These differences are evidence not of culture "loss" but of an active generation of culture—that capacity of each new generation to build communal values and character, to respond to individual and communal challenges, in ways they deem appropriate. Their children and grandchildren have remained on the reservation rather than moving away. They have built deep relationships in lives together with other Pima community members and one or two nonmembers. They choose among jobs, residences, pastimes, foods, and education in ways that facilitate a happy and good life on the rez, within their family and relationships, and in psychologically (individually) satisfying ways. Yes, there are elements they would change; but for what culturally "intact" group is that not true?

Family life is a human universal. Whether biological or fictive, nuclear or extended, family relations are the breathed air of social life, the first, most important way we interface with the world around us from birth. Generalizing the impact of this set of relations is treacherous terrain since the known diversity of global family forms and functions is large and growing. But its basic purpose to enculturate each new member, and by extension each new generation, into the most important ideas, forms of communication, values, and practices of a community is simply elemental.

Indigeneity communities are *generated* as each new member learns to value and participate in the community, each one having investment in and taking ownership in the group. Their enculturation begins immediately and continues throughout life, and the degree to which each individual perpetuates old forms or generates new ones will be a measure of the flexibility and self-determinative capacity of that community at any given point in time. Pima individualism is, therefore, as essential as Pima communalism. This is not to say that Indigenous peoples are *equally* individualistic as certain caricatures of Western individualism. It is to emphasize that selfish and self-serving motivations are a natural element of human life and must be nurtured and controlled in particular ways.

============

CHAPTER 3

Representation

Few social science topics are as manifold as "representation." This term can refer to a semiotic process, the role of a proxy, a depiction in visual or lyrical form, a claim as to fact, and a governmental office. The term invokes questions of authenticity, rights, and strategy. Representation makes possible things like stigma, prejudice, marginalization, and exploitation, but it is also a necessary part of group expression, cohesion, and learning. Finally and evident with rising globalism, representation has increasingly material effects. Indigenous peoples seek the access and authority available through representational form, be they local and specific or global and pan-Indigenous. The representational effort of Indigenous peoples to participate in this marketplace of meanings is not just a reflective or performative process alone. It can be constitutive.[1]

The historical representations of the Pima are fairly consistent in portraying them as successful farmers, as valuable guides and allies against the Apache, and as open to business relations, religious conversion, and cooperative coexistence with Anglo settlers. Until the middle of the nineteenth century (even after the Civil War), the Pimas' military and agricultural expertise made them essential allies, first to the Mexican and then to the American government. A number of O'odham leaders came to represent the Pima to the colonists and are named in historical accounts. One important example was Antonio Azul, general of the indomitable Pima-Maricopa Confederation (Dobyns 1989). But war, disease, and famine transformed those once economically prosperous communities of the Sonoran Desert. Pimas were starving and marginalized from the mid-nineteenth century to the mid-twentieth. Dobyns identifies a significant transition when, in 1908, former general Azul died, passing on his legacy to his son Antonito, who would become "chief of the Pima. The title, less resounding than 'general,' reflected the ebbing of Pima power since the time 50 years earlier when the Confederation had been a real military force (Dobyns 1989, 74).

By the mid- and late twentieth century, Pimas appeared in representational accounts far less often. A number of exceptional individuals were recognized: war heroes like J. R. Thomas, Sam Thomas, and Ira Hayes; rarely recorded women leaders and matriarchs, like Anna Moore Shaw (Shaw 2016) and Tohono O'odham Maria Chona (Underhill 1936); Rodney Lewis, a UCLA-trained lawyer who became general counsel for the Gila River Indian Community (GRIC) and worked for decades to secure the community's rightful water allotment; and a number of political and business leaders, like William R. Rhodes, who served the GRIC as a chief judge, lieutenant governor, tribal council member, and governor. But many Pima were angered and offended by other news representations (Smith-Morris 2006b; Smith-Morris and Epstein 2014) in which their disease statistics, poverty, and crime come to dominate the representational narrative.

The meager and often negative characterizations of native communities prior to the mid-1900s reflect a common prejudicial failure of dominant society to value subaltern groups or to give native authors the opportunity to express themselves to a larger audience. Anthropologists and historians made important contributions, of course, but those representations reflected Western categorical definitions of the Other and priorities for what was, and was not, recorded. The style of salvage ethnography, in which native peoples were viewed as a disappearing group, was typical of cultural representations well into the 1970s. Culture appeared as static, categorical, and in decline.[2] Only as Native Americans claimed some influence over these representations—either by representing themselves or by working with non-natives to alter the dominant ethic of engagement and representation—would the greater picture of Indigenous intellect, aspirations, and vision become clear to others.

In this chapter I draw a limited and community-focused line around a vast subject area. Other volumes dealing solely with the topic of representation offer readers a catalog, history, and impact assessment of representations employed by and foisted upon Indigenous peoples. I am more interested in how we might decolonize representations of Indigenous communalism and communities. For my discussion, I focus on three things. First, I consider the *authoritative* aspects and impacts of representation, being careful to differentiate authoritative from nonauthoritative forms of representation (Hodgson 2002; Tania Li 2000; Werbner 2002; Sylvain 2002). I examine public representational offices at Gila River—specifically, elected Tribal Council members and other elected or consensually supported public figures who are allowed to speak for the community. I am particularly interested in the authority given to these representatives and how Indigenous peoples often have to accommodate Western modes of representation in order to access and negotiate power. As part of this discussion, I consider some implications of written legal codes for traditionally orally governed and relational peoples. Second, I address Indigenous knowledge(s) and the ways that knowledge is represented in contemporary debates. In particular, I am concerned with the language of "ownership" of knowledge—a formulation that poorly represents Indigenous approaches to and purposes for their traditional knowledge. The concept of "alienable" content privileges Western and capitalistic ideals of commodification and exchange, a representational restriction impacting Indigenous possibilities for self-determination. And finally, in a third section I evaluate the body and Indigenous genetics as subjects of representational work. Body representations, including ones on the surface and underneath the surface, have become increasingly vulnerable to non-Indigenous manipulation and messaging in this age of genetic medicine.

AUTHORITY AND REPRESENTATION

There are no chiefs or rulers but there are highly respected and influential men and women referred to today as "elders" or "the old people." Recognition and authority come not just with age but through the respect that is gained over a lifetime by a person who does the right thing by him or herself, and by their own people.
—Gaynor Macdonald, *Two Steps Forward, Three Steps Back*

One cannot understand the role of an elected representative at Gila River without addressing the expectations of authority figures common to Indigenous groups. As with the Australian Aboriginal people described above by Gaynor Macdonald, traditional forms of authority at Gila River are typically reserved for "servants of their people" (Boldt 1993, 120).

Traditional leadership among the O'odham was village-based. According to the early nineteenth-century work of Ruth Underhill, villages were inhabited by relatives, usually on the father's side, among whom a leader of sorts was "elected" to settle disputes and lead ceremonies ([1941] 2000, 33). Leaders could pass down their knowledge to sons, but if the village did not approve of the headman's choice, "they asked him to teach someone else" (35). Other men led in warfare, hunting, and spiritual affairs according to their skills, age, and village support. And relationships—rather than offices—created conduits across which all of the political, social, spiritual, and economic functions of the community would occur.[3]

Also common to Indigenous forms of leadership and authority are intergenerational responsibilities. Elders and other representatives of the community are expected to maintain proper relations with the ancestors, expanding not only their social responsibilities but their obligations to enact long-term and sustainable policies on behalf of the people. Wendy Brady, the first Aboriginal person in Australia awarded a PhD, explains how "the sovereign Indigenous nation is formed through the ancestral and communal relationship. Unlike the sovereign of the European nation, authority does not reside in one figurehead and is not exercised downwards through layers of ever-declining levels of power. In the Indigenous nation, each individual is part of the fabric of both authority and power that is interdependent on the other" (Brady 2007, 142).

But soon after their arrival in the late eighteenth century, the Spanish would appoint a representative for the Pima, giving them authority to speak for and to larger groups or "towns" of O'odham (Underhill 1936, 36). So quite early on, the traditional structures of authority (and prestige) were upset. These colonial patterns are well known to have disturbed the balance of social status and authority among Indigenous groups, destabilizing traditional forms of education, social control, and leadership.

Today, and since the adoption of the Pima-Maricopa Indian Community constitution in 1936, representatives are elected to serve three-year terms on the Tribal Council. Traditional priorities such as relational work and consensus decision making are still intact. Any elected representative at Gila River is expected to not only consider and evaluate the issue at hand, including various sets of data that speak to that issue for her or his immediate and exigent opinion, but also decide when and how to engage the perspectives and opinions of others. This is a heavy burden for elected representatives at Gila River and across Indian Country where laws and economic factors are exponentially more complex than generations ago. Relational obligations are more diffuse and intense for Pima Tribal Council members than the specific duties of a dominant-society elected office, which garners more respect *as* an office on its own merits.

The more institutionalized form of representation in larger, democratic nation-states, where for example office holders must adhere to a code of ethics and fidelity but are not expected to achieve consensus within their home communities, has not been fully adopted at Gila River. Nor have constitutional governments entirely transformed other reservation communities because both scale and Indigenous values demand it. For enormous nation-states, elected offices themselves are a necessary adjustment to scale. These societies are simply too large for personal relationships between elected officials and each person they represent. But even Rousseau addressed the dangers of anonymity, nonparticipation, and corruption in *Social Contract*. He insisted that political liberty *presupposes* universal participation and that representation (rather than participation) would be "fatal to liberty" (Pitkin 1969, 6).

I imagine Rousseau would be pleased with the syncretic work of elected officers in tribal communities: those who remain closely tied to the subjective, experiential, and local qualities of life across their communities. Indigenous representatives are more often judged by the degree to which they embody (or are perceived to embody) these representational ideals. Indeed, those being represented maintain *greater* expectations for their elected representatives to embody not just what is "typical" of the group but the *best* qualities in the group.

In small-scale communities, any protection or privacy afforded to elected representatives by distance and scale is much less. So while it is often a rare surprise when politicians at the U.S. federal level are caught in corrupt behaviors, it can be well or more quickly known across reservation communities.[4] Just in recent years, there have been oustings of a Seminole Tribal Council chairman, a Northern Cheyenne chairman, and four Winnebago councilmembers. No matter how few community members fully embody community ideals, elected or chosen representatives are nevertheless expected to behave as ideal *individuals* and to promote the best interests of the community. And while this can be said of most elected representatives, the scale of Indigenous communities typically promotes greater scrutiny of representatives' actions.

Now, unlike representative leaders who can be influenced or removed from office, written representations can transcend time and place, remaining powerful long after they were first created. For colonized Indigenous peoples, written representations can create not just legal conditions that perpetuate colonial era injustices; they risk relational abuses in the disregard of humans' and communities' needs to adapt and change over time.

Innumerable examples of the representational immortality of written words exist in the treaties, court opinions, and laws passed during the colonial era but still influencing contemporary relations. For example, I draw from the work of J. Kēhaulani Kauanui, a Native Hawaiian and professor of anthropology and American studies at Wesleyan University in Middleton, Connecticut. Kauanui has helped document the continued battle for sovereignty being waged by Native Hawaiians. For this group's 1.8 million acres of native territories, there was never any exchange of money, never a treaty, and no case law. The lands were given (in written law) to the United States in 1889. For Native Hawaiians to win federal recognition, especially through the 2008 Akaka Bill proposed to Congress by Senator Daniel Akaka (D-HI): "Hawaii could never have casinos, never have criminal and civil jurisdiction, never petition the secretary of the Interior Department to take land into trust and never be able to make land claims under the 1790 Non-Intercourse Act" (Kauanui 2008). Under this agreement, Native Hawaiians would remain marginalized, impoverished, and weakened in their capacities as a community, all stemming from a decision made in 1790. Even as the gross violations of human and communal rights of the colonial era have been recognized, the power structures formed by that era remain securely in place. Not correction and certainly not reparation or reconciliation (see, e.g., Echo-Hawk 2016) is easily won. Federal representations of individual ownership and capitalist privilege (rather than relational priorities and stewardship of nature) remain dominant.

Note the representational quality of the written word—standing in for an agreement between parties or as the record of an historical truth—and the authority of that written document to immortalize the moment of its creation.

This idea of a representation having agency, or of a representative acting for others, is actually a recent idea, having begun to emerge only in the Middle Ages. In Latin, *repraesentare* means to make present or manifest or to present again. In her introduction to a collection on the topic of political representation, Pitkin explained that by the seventeenth century representation had become a political concept "worth fighting for . . . as one of the universal 'Rights of Man'" (1969, 4). The process of legally documenting an agreement—while intending to represent something agreed between parties in relationship with one another—can actually obliterate the role of relationship and negotiation. For relational communities, the written representation stands for a relationship but does not replace it.

The process whereby interactional obligations change from a commitment based on personal knowledge and trust between speakers to one of role-based obligations codified by the words on the page seems an inescapable dilemma of scale and complexity. Yet Indigenous groups need representations that better reflect these priorities and offer the possibility of improving their positions rather than accepting a disadvantaged status quo. For example, from a relational perspective, Indigenous communities might aim for representations that can be (re) ratified by contemporary parties. It is an approach to legal and political representation well aligned with Rousseau's emphasis on participatory governance, if not also a smaller scale than contemporary "mass, megatonnage and megalopolis" (Pitkin 1969, 6). This aim is very much related to Indigenous peoples' heritage of oral, rather than written, histories and a fundamentally different worldview about knowledge. As David Martinez has explained in reference to the Dakota, "knowledge is contained by people in social roles that were and are meaningful to the tribe: medicine, storytelling, ceremony, hunting, warfare, vision, and dream" (2009 153). These differences are not simple elements of literacy; they are poorly understood ontological differences between settler nations and Indigenous groups (e.g., Ramos 2012).

Although much more could be said about authority and representation for Indigenous peoples (see, e.g., Gomez 2016; Schroedel and Aslanian 2017), I have focused here on the relational and intergenerational obligations tied to people, offices, and written expressions that (claim to) represent Indigenous peoples. These are variables most important to the Indigenous communal process, which demands respect not only for relational priorities but also for intergenerational continuity. Indigenous peoples therefore hold different positionalities vis-à-vis written and nonrelational forms of representation, including laws and treaties based on past agreements made from different positions. Although Indigenous peoples are increasingly successful in navigating Western forms of law and writing, taking best advantage of a global shift toward humanitarian ethics, Indigenous ways of being, including relational priorities to living and ancestral beings, still need better options.

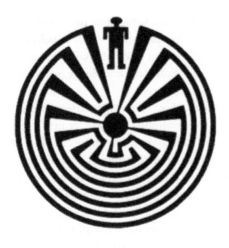

Figure 6. The man in the maze symbol is shared by the Akimel and the Tohono O'odham, and represents man's journey through life.

REPRESENTING COMMUNAL KNOWLEDGE

As more Indigenous peoples have gained the knowledge, language, and credentials they needed to advocate for themselves in courts and in the international media, the concept of communal knowledge has come to the fore. Neither international nor state laws have been particularly good at representing communal Indigenous knowledge in ways that protect it from exploitation. In particular, the concept of "alienability," something fairly essential to Western legal structures through patent and property laws, suggests a form of possession foreign to many Indigenous groups (Moreton-Robinson 2011). If something is "alienable," it can be removed from one person and transferred or sold to another. The term typically refers either to objects or entities or to the right to control certain objects or entities, but patent law and intellectual property laws are not easily applied to communal forms of knowledge.

The concept of intellectual property is not foreign to Indigenous peoples. As Conklin (2002) has explained, Indigenous peoples' knowledge of the natural environment within the territories of their heritage is one such entity. But to defend their traditional knowledge, Indigenous groups have had to define it as a matter of "property" subject to personal "ownership," concepts that are somewhat antagonistic to Indigenous ways of thinking. Alienability is the authoritative frame limiting what is even possible for Indigenous self-determination. Again, it was Conklin who explained that privileged knowledge about, say, medicinal plants or sacred rituals is not necessarily restricted to certain persons within a community; it can be widely shared among members. But this knowledge is nevertheless a "precious possession" (1057) that both is private and should, according to doctrines on collective rights, be inalienable to the collective. The sharing of such knowledge, either with community members or with outsiders, is not intended to transfer that privileged possession; subsequent publication or use of that knowledge—whether in ethnographic, pharmaceutical, or political contexts—poses a complicated problem. And current international patent laws are poor instruments for protecting Indigenous traditional knowledge (see Mead 2002 for an insightful discussion of Maori experience).

As the assumptions of Western legal approaches to knowledge are reconsidered by Indigenous scholars, what constitutes communal knowledge may itself be changing. In recent decades, Native American communities have established creative legal frameworks for research within their community's boundaries (Smith-Morris 2007; Kovach 2015). Research is a process by which scientists evaluate phenomena in the world to suggest the order, causality, meanings, and other explanations of those phenomena. When phenomena are social and the data are gathered from human subjects, the phenomena in question are often deemed significant only to the extent that they *represent* a large population. The researcher's role vis-à-vis this type of communally owned information, if not also the representations that emerge from that research, has come under increasing scrutiny. And the history of tribal-anthropologist research relationships has vacillated in step with federal Indian policy (Canby 2014). In 1886, the *Illustrated Police News* and *New York Herald* published a story about Matilda Coxe Stevenson's work with Zuni. She (like Frank Cushing) is known to have insisted that natives provide her with information for her research, under the justification of salvage ethnography. The article was titled "Cowed by a Woman: A Craven Red Devil Weakens in the Face of a Resolute White Heroine" (Parezo 1993, 46). Somewhat less presumptuous was Muriel Painter, also a painstaking ethnographer. Her work among the Yoeme (Yaqui) from the 1920s to the 1960s produced such detailed and accurate descriptions that some Yoeme apparently consulted with her on proper ways of conducting ceremonial (especially Easter) activities, correct adornments, and even dance patterns (Parezo 1993). Painter collaborated and coauthored works with Native Americans, acknowledging their ownership and authorship of the information on which she could base a career. It was a Navajo community project at Crownpoint, New Mexico, in the same era—the 1950s—that would help germinate the discipline of applied anthropology. This project by Flathead tribe member D'Arcy McNickle began with a focus on health issues but expanded to how communities can and do make larger economic development decisions. Improvements in the rigor, value, and ethics of applied anthropology have been made as more native peoples have taken up the work themselves.

Although in the Western industrial complex we recognize corporate and trade secrets and can even conceptualize group ownership of patented ideas, the secret-sacred cultural knowledge of Indigenous peoples is not well represented by (or in) Western laws. To become ownable, such knowledge must be transformed into legally precise documentation and given an individual or corporate owner.

Secret-sacred knowledge passed down orally through generations has also been recognized—with difficulty—in a growing body of law such as the Native Title Act of Australia and the World Trade Organization's 1994 Agreement on Trade Related Aspects of Intellectual Property Rights (Ragavan 2001; Sand 2002). But the ideological and legal contests over cultural knowledge still stumble over whether these are represented as individual or communal rights (Rimmer 2015; Jackson and Warren 2005).

Native American communities have called for change. When Beverly Becenti-Pigman, chairman of the Navajo Nation Institutional Review Board, spoke to a gathering of southwestern U.S. tribal representatives, she summed up an important concern: "We get the impression researchers view the rez as a land of opportunity" (Jadrnak 2006). Not much later, Champagne noticed that few anthropology graduate students were working on native issues or with native U.S. communities. More important, Native American community members have had greater opportunity to lead anthropological applied work and research themselves. This improving capacity helps tribes to gain control over and to extract greater benefits from research in Indian Country (Champagne and Goldberg 2005; Cochran et al. 2008; Wallerstein and Duran 2006; Darling et al. 2015). Native communities are no longer passive recipients of "outside experts" but balance the dueling priorities of, on the one hand, the sanctity of cultural heritage and privacy and, on the other, legal and political needs to demonstrate cultural vitality, longevity, stewardship, and even membership.

Ultimately for research, the question of "Who owns cultural knowledge?" is being reclaimed by tribes. For example, the Native Nations Institute at the University of Arizona has developed a "network of colleagues and collaborators" to address "the need for tribes to drive their data agendas through practicing Indigenous data sovereignty and governing their information."[5] Indigenous communities and groups like the one at the University of Arizona increasingly face questions: Is knowledge something that rests with an individual, and is it alienable? Or can ownership be something shared across people, even across generations, such that the knowledge is inalienable? If, as has been argued, culture is recognized as a shared event, then knowledge of that culture must belong in some measure to the group as a whole, indivisible and inalienable. Ultimately, framing these issues in terms of ownership may be a misrepresentation.

REPRESENTATION AND RACE—COMMUNAL GENETICS

For a third view on representation, I consider the types of representation that our bodies provide. Bodily characteristics can be representational of an inner identity, health, and/or intentions of a person. Inscriptions upon the body, for example, henna or tattoo images, expand the representational capacity of our physical forms. These representational forms are individual—in the physical manifestation on a particular body—as well as communal or cultural—in the symbols used and what they convey to the bearers and to their various readers. Whether for beauty, remembering, protest, or simply the physical experience of emblazoning a message onto one's skin, body manipulations like these open up wide possibilities for representation.

With scientific advances in genetics, inscriptions *within* the human body are now being read and represented in astounding new ways. Not only do companies like 23andMe offer to reveal clues of an individual's genetic heritage (including any lurking disease proclivities), but these technologies can also expose family- or population-level patterns that individuals may not wish to learn (Annas and Elias 2014; Wynn and Chung 2017). For Indigenous peoples, whose blood quantum membership rules (where present) mean that members will share some genetic features, a community's genetic code—not just the individual's— is vulnerable to the representations and interpretations of outsiders (e.g., Hsueh et al. 2017).

The Pimas have experience with this type of unwelcome genetic representation. Scientists have used biotechnology and epidemiological prediction to describe the Pima genetic code and predict disease rates, especially for diabetes (e.g., Hanson et al. 2015). In an age of genetic medicine, diabetes has become somewhat of a scar at the molecular level, a representation of their health about which Pimas have expressed resentment and frustration (see, e.g., Smith-Morris 2006b; Wailoo and Pemberton 2006). A disease caused historically and economically by colonial events is, instead, represented as the result of *faulty genetics* and *individual behaviors*. From the Pima perspective those genetics allowed them to thrive in the desert environment where others (namely European settlers) could not.

I have explored the Pimas' collective experience of illness in greater depth in other writings (Smith-Morris 2006b). Scars of hardship are a reminder of these shared experiences and become emblematic of a continuing shared identity and interest. Illness can form one type of communal scar, whether it emerges from a genetic cause or from a shared biological exposure. In fact, illness always creates a community out of its victims—sufferers from leprosy, patients diagnosed with x-disease, and the victims of the Tuskegee experiments create communities via their shared experiences. The fact that the Pima share what James Neel called a "thrifty gene"—which turned out to be a collection of inherited traits relevant to metabolic disorders—is a representational scar that points directly back to colonization and the dramatic and swift change in subsistence strategy colonization forced (Neel 1962; Ayub et al. 2014).

It was the Pimas' high recorded rates of diabetes that brought them to the attention of the National Institute of Diabetes and Digestive and Kidney Diseases (NIDDKD)—a federal research organization that based its operations in

Phoenix to be near this community. The decades-long relationship that Pimas had with the NIDDKD as research subjects significantly impacted not only those subjects who participated in research but the community as a whole. The Gila River Indian Community Council, in particular, has experienced the pros and cons of this attention. They have had more experience with research and contracted health care than perhaps any other tribe in the United States. But for them, the payoff to this research and health care dipped below its perceived costs. At least some key members of the community and council hoped that by reducing the research presence on the reservation, community members might rely less on biomedical fixes (e.g., medications) for this epidemic. And this communal sentiment prompted a closure of the NIDDKD offices on the reservation and several other changes in clinical programming.

Miguel is college-educated man whose narratives about Pima lifeways and history, quoted in chapter 1, are often emotional and strongly opinionated. I met him early in my time at Gila River, and we have become both collaborators and friends over the years. When he speaks about diabetes, he can recite both the genetic and environmental factors in its etiology, is familiar with the rates of this disease at Gila River and across Indian Country, and is knowledgeable and direct about the decades-long relationship of the National Institutes of Health diabetes researchers to the tribe: "My theory is that when they shut down the river many, many years ago we were forced to stray away from fish and fresh vegetables and given high fat things and forced to make up frybread with lard. Just a whole change of diet that caused it back then. We had to work out. We go from eating fresh fish and fresh vegetables and all of a sudden you get canned goods, lard." He's right. Despite being a symbol of pan-Indian foodways, frybread is an invention of commodity days. The government pantry offered salt, flour, baking powder, and lard, so Pimas and other Native Americans all over the country fashioned this into their daily bread. At Gila River, they eat plate-sized frybread or huge chumuth tortillas; in the northern Pueblos, the same ingredients were made into loaves and cooked in outdoor ovens; the Seminoles made a smaller disk of dough and fried it in oil. The effect of their decades-long dependency on commodities is, indeed, a major factor in Pima diabetes.

Arnold, a thirty-five-year-old unemployed man with an eighth-grade education, has a similar perspective. He too can reproduce an explanation of geneticist James Neel's "thrifty genotype hypothesis" without a flaw. It is the explanation given to him his whole life by educators and clinicians:

> I think it is, just because of the tests that they've done prove that Pimas are more—well, the explanation I was given, and it made sense what they said—was that Pimas were just generally thin people because they ran and walked back in the day, everywhere they went. And everything they ate was healthy. And then when they got exposed to the lards and the sugars, that their bodies

were so used to making do with the little they had, when they got these things that had so much of it, that's what made them big. Normally they were thin people but their body just overloaded on the bad stuff and that's why they got big. So I think, yeah, they can't help it because it's in their body make-up.

But other Pimas, even ones who recognize the role of diet in diabetes, attribute the epidemic here to a more generalized trauma in their tribe's history. Dillan was a twenty-eight-year-old warehouse worker when he responded to a poster advertisement recruiting participants for a study about diabetes at Gila River. Having earned his GED and working full-time, he had a solid income to care for his own family of four and to provide some financial help to his mother, who lived on her own in another district. His mother had diabetes, and his father had it before his death several years before we met. Although his dad ignored the medicines and advice he got about diabetes, his mother tried to keep up with a growing inventory of pills, including insulin shots. Dillan, like most Pimas, had years of firsthand observation of this disease and its ravages on the body. His father had died before the outward signs were particularly visible, but his mom had already had two toes amputated and was developing vision problems. When I asked him to talk about the disease and its particular meaning for Pimas, he said he knew it was "from the salt and sugar and overeating" but then added, "I believe that it was from way back when we lost our river and a lot of people started stressing out and all they did was eat. And that's how they started getting diabetes. Then everybody started inheriting it through their bloodline."

And finally, there are those, like Virgil, who recognize threats in every corner: history, genetics, foods, stress, talking about it too much, and personal choices. When I asked him where he thought the diabetes epidemic came from, he asked me, "What *doesn't* give Pimas diabetes?"

I know everybody has it, like Anglos, a lot of people, whatever. But for the Indians it was, what didn't give it to them? We didn't get that intentionally but it's there now. But now I think the society is not encouraging [them] but [instead] giving them more grease, more sugar, stuff like that. Get it worse, whatever! But when we did get it, it was like "oh yeah, give me more sugar. Give me more grease" or whatever. Yeah, or if you talk about it too much, yeah, that's part of that too. Like I say, the water went out and they couldn't do what they used to do before. And it's probably what made it worse, probably part of the reason, the whole life thing. Everything has a reason for something and stress going through you, man, gotta eat some more.

Not just because of its epidemic proportion but because of its character as representational scar, diabetes at Gila River can quite literally be seen as a community issue, not an individual one. A collective response is therefore an appropriate if not a natural one to a collective problem.

Puneet Sahota, a physician and anthropologist, studied the reaction of an unnamed group of Native Americans in the Southwest to being told their genetics put them at high risk for diabetes. Their responses ranged from depression and fear to shame and hopelessness (closely related to what Kozak 1997 called "surrender"). Sahota also collected a number of narratives, like those above, that described diabetes as a scar representing a history of colonization, losses of land and water, and the erosion of traditional foods and practices under the assimilating pressures of poverty. Sahota wrote, "Their comments about their 'genes' and 'bodies' are linked to their narratives about the collective and painful history of their tribe. Their references to 'our bodies' and shared 'genes' also reveal their view that tribal members share a collective ethnic identity based in their bodies/genes . . . their group self-perceptions" (2012, 833).

Pressure on individuals within these genetic-patient communities—whether to reduce their symptoms, to contain their infectious behavior, or to raise heathier children despite a disease-producing context—are also felt collectively. At Gila River, these pressures come in the forms of encouragement, funding, education, motivational classes, incentive programs, and research. Pimas are not incarcerated or forced into medical treatments, but there is a demoralizing and oppressive effect from epidemiological racism and from the mounting strategies to medicalize Pima lives. Refusal to participate in diabetes treatment or prevention activities defies pressures to change, no matter how well intentioned. For example, these are the behaviors of Pimas who attend some biomedical appointments but follow instructions and advice selectively, do not share complete health details, and use medications differently than prescribed (Smith-Morris 2006b). This resistance is certainly part of native survivance (Stromberg 2006a; Powell 2002) against domination by non-native ideologies, including biomedical ones.

Finally, wherever epidemic levels of diabetes have been present for multiple generations and where both genetic and gestational (or intrauterine) factors contribute to younger and younger ages at diagnosis, people will come to believe that the disease is a permanent and nearly unavoidable part of the community (Smith-Morris 2006a). The high rates of disease are attributable as much to their history of colonization, their loss of groundwater, their traditional lifestyle based on farming, and the dilemmas of development as to their bad eating habits and failure to exercise (Smith-Morris and Epstein 2014). Personal responsibility for disease is a biomedical paradigm that, while present in many Gila River community members to varying degrees, remains an issue of contention and power.

Of course the vast majority of treatment for this condition occurs individually, but there remains a communal undercurrent of resistance—not only to treatments but also to seeking or receiving a diagnosis and to monochromatic representations of their community centered on this (or another) health issue.

Pima resistance to biomedical-centric representations disperses responsibility for diabetes to the Tribal Council, to health care practitioners, to colonial and postcolonial disenfranchisement, to genetics, and to the overwhelming sum of these factors. Representational scars merit this response. The individualist, disease-focused framework of the biomedical worldview is simply, and grossly, inadequate for acknowledging this disease at Gila River.

REPRESENTING INDIGENOUS DIVERSITY

The process of representation has central implications for Indigenous communalism because it is such an important communicative and symbolic device. If they are to cohere and survive, communities must be able to define and represent themselves, even unto themselves. Indigenous peoples clearly excel in the internal representational work of community. But they have also begun to exert more control over literary and public representations of their communities and to demand respect for Indigenous relational and intergenerational priorities in those representations.

Indigenous communalism was only weakly represented in the salvage ethnography typical of the twentieth century. My goal for this chapter has been to expose some of the representational limits and possibilities with specific and day-to-day examples. Rather than a static and dying culture languishing under its poverty or acculturating into dominant global forms, as it appears in classic ethnographies, Gila River is shown here as a dynamic and creative community resisting the ideological assumptions of governance, law, and health (see also chapter 5). Community members strategize to represent themselves as good Indians (good Pimas) in a variety of ways, traditional and nontraditional. And the very diversity of their strategies belies the limits of static ethnological representations.

Scholars help decolonize representations of Indigenous communalism in several ways. First, by making fewer claims as to universal or structural patterns within society, the language of ethnography and cultural study has become more descriptive and less proscriptive. This distinction does not necessarily preclude theoretical or comparative engagement with Indigenous communities, but it does insist upon local and specific units of analysis. Second, representations of Indigenous communities should be aggressive and meticulous in their questioning of ideological assumptions. I have addressed ideas of knowledge, ownership, and democratic representation, but these are mere introductions to the expository and corrective work of Indigenous scholars and activities. Legal scholars and historians, in particular, will have to work with culture scholars and artists (all Indigenous and non-Indigenous) to dismantle the settler-colonial ideologies and their representations.

Representation has been the third of four elements in Indigenous communalism. In the fourth element, which is the human capacity for hybridity between the values of individualism and communalism, I grapple most earnestly with some of the issues that challenge Indigenous rights to sovereignty, namely individual autonomy, heterogeneity within communities, and conflicts between individual human rights and communal/collective rights.

=============

Hybridity

No man is an island, entire of itself; every man is a piece of the continent, a part of the main. If a clod be washed away by the sea, Europe is the less, as well as if a promontory were, as well as if a manor of thy friend's or of thine own were: any man's death diminishes me, because I am involved in mankind.
—John Donne, *No Man Is an Island—A Selection from the Prose*

We are all islands—in a common sea.
—Anne Morrow Lindbergh, *Gift from the Sea*

Growing up in the shadow of poverty, alcoholism, and periodic violence, Michael was the fourth of eight children. He was raised until the age of eight in his parents' home, enjoying the company of older and younger siblings and being known as the best runner among the kids. As a child he and his brothers wandered around in the back yard and later out away from the houses into the desert, where he could challenge his older brother and sisters to races. "I had stamina!," which he said always brought victory. When he described these running races to me and the feeling of speed and strength in his legs with only the mountains in front of him and his rival falling behind him, his pride and nostalgia for youth almost overwhelmed him.

But when his parents' arguments became violent, Michael and the older children were moved into his aunt's house. A custody battle took place in the tribal court system, but Michael wasn't aware of the details—only that his parents would sometimes be gone for days at a time and that both had spent time in jail. Whenever he saw or spoke to them on the phone, they insisted they wanted their kids back. In his younger years he had spent nights or weeks with his aunt when his parents didn't come home. Now, he said, it was just a permanent arrangement.

When he reached eighth grade, Michael was still riding to the public middle school by bus with his cousins and other kids from the reservation. It picked him up almost two hours before school started and brought him home about ninety minutes afterward. School was pleasant enough and Michael was passing all his subjects except math. But he was very quiet in school, finding that the non-Indian kids would always satisfy the teachers' requests before he had to. Teachers rarely called on him, he thinks now, because they knew it made him uncomfortable. And the lack of involvement grew over the years into a pattern of back-row non-participation. Combining this generally mute experience in class with his failure to turn in homework, Michael had to attend summer school after sixth and seventh grades. By the time he moved out of his parents' house, he was already on shaky ground to reach that major reservation milestone: graduation from eighth grade.

Michael told me he had exactly four friends in middle school. Not that he had four best friends, but that there were exactly four kids with whom he interacted in any way. It seemed like a small number, but knowing Michael's extremely quiet personality, I wasn't surprised. Not having shadowed him in school, I couldn't tell whether this mild degree of isolation was a result of Michael's own self-imposed separation or a pattern among Indian kids. I suspect it was a combination of both.

Middle school is a period of enormous social and relational challenges anyway. The cultural and economic differences between reservation kids and non-Indian kids are almost insurmountable. Michael had the added stress and distraction of his changing family environment. So to have four good friends providing consistency across that transition was a fairly substantial positive in his ledger of life. And he did make it through eighth grade.

Some Pima families throw huge parties for their graduating eighth-graders, with dozens of extended kin from all over the reservation showing up with food and presents. Michael's celebration was nothing like that. His aunt bought him a cake, which he ate with his siblings and cousins. And his mother brought him a number 6 from McDonald's a few weeks later. Eighth-grade graduation is celebrated on the reservation because it is broadly recognized as a not-inevitable achievement. So that could have been the end of this window onto Michael's reservation childhood. A majority of Pima kids stop schooling at eighth grade or soon after and begin working and having their own children, sometimes more slowly, sometimes more quickly. But partly thanks to his aunt's encouragement, partly due to the fact that Michael's four friends were continuing, Michael went to ninth grade. His aunt had gone to high school for several months, then got pregnant and quit. His older cousins had either never gone or also quit before tenth grade, spending their time instead on the living room sofa, plugged in to computer games or the TV. Many of them graduated to more dangerous and illegal activities like shoplifting, smoking pot, or selling drugs, which were things Michael was too introverted to think desirable.

Michael's aunt was like many other parents on the reservation: loath to scold children when they themselves had behaved similarly as youth. In a conversation with me about parenting, another Pima man put it this way: "It's more that the parents don't know to tell them. They've never experienced it. And it goes back to they've never experienced it themselves. If you haven't experienced it, how can you practice it? I think a lot of parents, they just have kids and they're not prepared for them. They're pregnant [too young] and they were never taught how to raise kids." Michael's father and aunt learned parenting from their own parents, whom Michael described as "drunks." My impression was that his grandparents were heavy but nonviolent drinkers who never had any money. The kids learned to find food and company on their own and had become "wild teenagers," as Michael described them. But Michael's aunt had settled down over the years, while Michael's father had not. His aunt settled down when she gave birth to a daughter with a heart defect. She quit the drugs and gave up the wilder people in her life. More than fifteen years later, in her thirties, she attended classes and got her GED. So by the time Michael and his siblings needed a new home, she had been stable for many years with a job cleaning at the casino. Knowing that the tribe would pay for it, she had even looked into classes at the local community college.

That information would prove useful to Michael, who became proud of his new home and of the turnaround his aunt had made in her life. Michael hoped to avoid some of the worst mistakes, like jail, bad relationships, violence, and drugs. His aunt simply told all the kids, "if you're going to do that, don't do it here." Michael didn't want to leave the house much, so he avoided a lot of trouble. Michael knows that it was his aunt's home environment, and his own personality, that made high school, much less college, a possibility. He simply preferred his aunt's home and school to some of the alternatives. It was his desire to be around his friends that got him from eighth grade to ninth, but it was his exposure to his Aunt's ideas, her steady income, and the atmosphere of a stable home that showed him a life other than what his own parents had shown him.

One night in conversation with this aunt, I glimpsed some of "his Aunt's ideas" and imagined a younger Michael hearing the same messages when he was a teenager. She said, "Indians won't be with Indians the rest of their lives. You have to interact with everybody else out there. You've got to get them ready for the real world. If you don't, you're going to fail because they're just not ready for it."

It is at this juncture that Michael's life illustrates an important aspect of hybridity. There are many ways that Michael might have pursued his life, many ways that would have been thoroughly Pima in character and squarely rooted in both reservation life and a family- and community-centered identity. He could have dropped out after (or even before) eighth grade, spending several years in idleness, substance abuse, or jail. He could have dropped out of school in favor of vocational training and earned a reasonable income that way. He might even have made his way with periodic odd jobs and living off the generosity of family and friends. All of these are common strategies among Pima youth, and lead many to happy, successful lives in the community.

But Michael's path involved an off-reservation high school because he liked it and he felt more comfortable attending school than in the company of his teenage cousins and friends who were experimenting with drugs and crime. Many might call Michael more individualistic for his drive to succeed in certain ways. But Michael's individuality and personality led him down a less common path. Even so, his individualism still fits comfortably within the universe of Pima lifeways and personalities. He experienced many of the challenges and rites of passage I know to be common at Gila River and many reservations (see Treuer 2012). This rite of passage can last up to ten years, sometimes more. And insofar as these experiences are common among Pima youth, they appear normal.

Even so, while so many personal and family challenges may be normative to reservation life, they are not comparable to the traditions in Pima heritage. Prior to their incorporation into Western schooling and wage labor, when Pimas reached an age of maturity, there were lessons in adulthood and tests of their skills. The abilities to hunt game or to work in the agricultural fields and irrigation ditches (for boys) or to prepare meals, keep a home, and care for children or elders (for girls) were scrutinized and evaluated by parents and elders (Shaw 2016). Couples were matched or found each other according to and in the hopes that these standards would make a happy life for them. There was work to be done, Apaches to watch out for, and relations to visit. Many of the same activities are prevalent today (although Apaches are now friends rather than mobile enemies), but they don't earn the prestige or cash that so define success according to contemporary standards.

I bring up these historical differences not to belabor the point of colonial trauma but to return the conversation to Pima individualism and to the choices made by individual Pimas under changing circumstances throughout their lives. Michael has made some uncommon choices and has now lived off reservation, but he is still immersed in his community and family, expressing his individualism without sacrificing his communal commitment. Michael's experience therefore adds an essential variable to a proper understanding of Indigenous communalism—the diversity of ways that community members will find to become and remain deeply connected, valued, and certainly "authentic" community members. Michael now holds a college degree and a well-paying job.

HYBRIDITY AND HUMAN COMMUNITY

The idea behind my first three foci in this book—belonging, generation, and representation—is fundamentally a Rousseauian lesson: that all societies are groups in which every individual has some personal investment. Communities are built such that individuals can feel that they belong. Members are generated to be "good" according to communal values and come to use or embody various representations of their larger community in its perpetuation.

I now add the most flexible element in this process, by which different members of the society can express their commitment to the group in varying ways over time. Because communalism and individualism are values informing choices and actions, they are enacted in impossibly diverse ways. They are not rigid typologies. Far from destroying individualism, communal forces inform and populate the myriad ways that individuals express themselves. Individualism is channeled into a limited set of prescribed models by each cultural community.

I turn, therefore, to the concept of hybridity. This commonly used idea is simply a mixture of two different elements. In my use of it, I am not suggesting that Indigenous peoples have some metaphysical character different from other humans. In fact, with hybridity I am referring to a universal human capacity to blend contradictory virtues into a meaningful but complex self-identity.[1] It is this capacity for both the individual and the communal together, the synergy of group and person, the *hybrid* experience within each of us, that ensures communalism is never without its interest in individuals. Hybridity also allows for changing priorities within a person's lifetime, making necessary adjustments to ancestral or traditional forms—as may be necessary when Indigenous peoples no longer have access to sacred spaces, to communal property, or to a viable living in a shared residential space. And last, hybridity between communalism and individualism is not only a human capacity but also a community capacity. As it does for individuals facing decisions across a lifetime, hybridity acknowledges the creative/productive process in which communities (re)generate themselves. As Lightfoot puts it, "Global Indigenous ultimately rests on a universal right to maintain difference" (2016, 202), a right intended to last into the future.

Despite historic presumptions about societal types—collectivist versus individualist societies—the scientific literature does not always bear out such extreme formulations. Even Melford Spiro was careful to express this hybridity in his ethnography of the kibbutz, a community built on equality among individuals, individual liberty, and the moral ideal of self-realization through labor:

> The group, in kibbutz culture, is not only a means to the happiness of the individual; the group and group processes are moral ends in their own right. This has three aspects. It means, first, that the interests of the individual must be subordinate to the interests of the group. When the needs of the individual and those of the group come into conflict, the individual is expected to abdicate his needs in favor of the group's. . . . A second aspect of the emphasis on the ethical value of the group involves the assumption that the individual's motivations will always be directed to the promotion of the group's interests,

as well as of his own. Behavior is expected to be characterized by *ezra hada-dit*, or mutual aid. This means that every member of the kibbutz is responsible for the welfare of every other member and for the welfare of the kibbutz as a whole, just as the kibbutz is responsible for the welfare of each individual. . . . The emphasis on the moral value of the group means, finally, that group living and group experiences are valued more highly than their individual counterparts. (Spiro 1956, 29–31)

Communalism even in this most collectivist form, an Israeli kibbutz, relies on the hybrid capacity of individuals to exist. Communities of many kinds will thrive or fail depending on the interest taken and investment made by individuals. For Spiro, communalism in the kibbutz is carefully nourished, trained up, and managed by the rules of membership and by the example of its leaders. Rather than antagonizing each other, the values of communalism and individualism work constantly and in fine increments toward balance. Societies around the world follow this same general pattern, developing ways to channel individuals into various models of success; individuals simultaneously learn and reason their way into values that situate them comfortably and correctly within the community. Although this situating may not be permanent or singular, once situated each member will reliably perform some minimum degree and form of communalist investment.

Consider the alternative briefly, as occurs for Indigenous peoples who are not given the privilege of hybridity, change, and internal heterogeneity. Only dominant cultures are allowed to be diverse and contradictory, while Indigeneity is expected to be "pure," of one mind and aesthetic, and easily identifiable (Sium, Desai, and Ritskes 2012, viii). Indigenous survivance, to borrow a term from Native American literary leaders (Powell 2002; Stromberg 2006a), means trying to resist the moral structuring of ideological colonialism. I am suggesting that ideologies of individualism are a key example of ideological colonialism that is active today (also consider the works of Krmpotich, Howard, and Knight 2016 and Howard 2018.).

This chapter contains some more overt claims about the moral bearings of communalism. Community building is about relationships and is negotiated, by nature. In Cheryl Mattingly's work among parents of children with cancer, this nature is "experimental" (2014); in Annemarie Mol's study of how we care for earth and each other through moral work called "tinkering" (Mol 2008; Mol, Moser, and Pols 2015). These authors emphasize that as individuals make decisions, they do not make a mathematical calculation of costs and benefits (Henrich 2002); they are doing moral work. For social animals like humans, communalism is therefore a moral subject, especially vis-à-vis human rights. The UN Universal Declaration of Human Rights was proclaimed in 1948, but dramatic additions came in 1966 when two more binding covenants—the International

Covenant on Economic, Social and Cultural Rights and the International Covenant on Civil and Political Rights—were passed. These latter two conventions speak directly to the social and collective rights of humans, without which individual rights cannot be fully achieved. In my estimation, these also form part of the bedrock on which the Declaration on the Rights of Indigenous Peoples was argued, written, and passed in 2007. As we tackle the most difficult questions of communalism—namely the potential for conflicts between extreme communal practices and individual human rights—we benefit from these institutionalized documents and the transnational moral consensus that produced them.

By the time I met Michael, as part of my second major research project at Gila River, he had met and married his wife; he had lived off the reservation for a few years but had returned and was raising his family there. They had no alcohol or drug problems, they expected their children to finish high school and consider college, and Michael hoped his kids would have the same fond memories of freedom and play in the desert that he had had. Both he, the college graduate, and his aunt, the one who dropped out of high school pregnant, recognize that there is variation in people's ability and desire to participate in Western-style education. Each learned skills and patterns to create their own individuality, to reach their own goals. And every other community member will do the same. Their stories are reminders that communalism and individualism are made up of the numberless decisions and moral choices.

Extremes of Communalism

To test the strength of one's commitment to this priority of communalism, consider a case *outside* of Native American communities. Certain cultural practices known to cause harm to individuals, but which represent important rites of commitment and morality within a community, test one's willingness to conform in ways not present at Gila River. Communalism is the reason why individual human rights violations can continue, as discussed in the 1995 Human Rights Watch publication "Playing the Communal Card." And these extreme forms therefore demand attention in a book like mine. Accordingly, I turn to one of the most contentious, emotional, and evocative issues of the late twentieth century: female genital cutting. I reiterate that this practice is not an Indigenous or tribal practice per se, but it does present us with an overt conflict between communal and individual rights. And for that reason I believe it is an important case to understand.

Female genital cutting (FC), the cutting and/or excision of portions of the female genitalia for nonmedical reasons, is a cultural practice that appears so strange and without merit to Western sensibilities that its very existence has called the practitioners' civility, rationality, even humanity into question (e.g., Cameron 2013). FC has been summarily denounced since 1997 by several international organizations, and great investments have been made in the forced or voluntary abandonment of this practice. And for decades it was targeted as a problem of "culture" and belief rather than the integrated system of meaning and practice it is (see, e.g., Merry 2003). But during the most recent decades, an international debate has grown over the rights and authority of local communities to set rules of morality and behavior for their own members. And it is this characteristic that justifies inclusion of FC here.

FC remains in practice in many communities around the world, and where it is resisted or condemned, the voices are *not* unanimous or unified. Instead, this issue illustrates at least two important questions for the present discussion: First, how committed are we to granting legitimacy to and protection for communal rights of self-determination? And second, should (and how can) an international community engage in cross-cultural dialogue about communal practices not their own or exert influence while retaining respect for communal self-determination?

It is well known that only if the practicing communities themselves decide to halt or modify their FC practices does change occur. For these reasons, FC is an important case to consider both ethnographically and with moral reasoning (that is, with judgment suspended, at least temporarily). As this is a case study for communalism, hyperindividualist readers may be challenged to engage deeply with this seemly incommensurable moral world and to temporarily suspend the assumptions of their own culture (if not also their own normative morality).[2] But that is the goal.

FC, like male genital cutting, is the practice (traditional in some cultures but, again, not at Gila River) of partially or totally removing the external genitalia for nonmedical reasons. FC is considered the most neutral term, although in much of the Western literature on FC the term "female genital mutilation" has also been used. "Mutilation" is an offensive term to those who practice FC since its implication is so negative, "tantamount to an accusation of evil intent" (Gruenbaum 2001, 3). (For help achieving cultural relativism, recall that a similar procedure is practiced almost universally on boy infants in America or that painful and medically unnecessary body modifications are common in all parts of the world.) Biomedicine calls these practices "mutilation" because healthy human tissue is removed for nonclinical purposes. Biomedicine is also concerned with short- and long-term threats to health that FC typically produces. But the biomedical "facts" are not so relevant as the social facts to my current conversation about individualist versus communalist values. The term "circumcision" is also inadequate for a different reason. While "circumcision" gives naming authority to the social aspects of the practice—the term being associated with a religious proscription and rite of passage—it literally means "to cut around" and thus directs itself to the foreskin of a human penis and not to the clitoris or parts of the vulva. The term "cutting" also helps decenter the bio-medical paradigm as authority for naming this practice.

FC, since it is medically unnecessary and can be quite dangerous, is a prime example of a costly collective norm. Among the concerns about FC are the pain and risk of the surgery, the lifelong health impacts for the girl, the economic context into which the girl was born and will likely live out her life, issues of parental responsibility for the raising of virtuous girls, the autonomy of individuals, the autonomy of cultural groups, and the relationship of individuals to their community. The consequences for this practice, and for any change to it, are therefore social, economic, and biological.

Failure to participate in FC or to have one's daughter undergo the procedure has historically harmed a girl's chances for marriage, particularly if this is her only route to normative adult roles and economic stability. In extreme cases, she could be completely isolated and unable to secure food or work. The stigma can be both personal and familial, there being great pressure on (and desire of) families to ensure that daughters are marriageable. So in societies where familial and social networks determine not only the woman's life chance but also the social and economic success of her relatives, the entire family is invested in each girl's FC because it impacts the livelihood of all its members.

Thus, several cultural reasons and norms (many stated, others more implied) stabilize the practice of FC against evolutionary odds. In some places it is not only socially adaptive but requisite, while in others less severe forms of FC have been accepted (Ahmadu 2000, 2017; Ahmadu and Shweder 2009).

Because of this circumstance, the FC debates are not just about individual choice but about community circumstances and self-determination. I draw particularly on the work of Ellen Gruenbaum and others who define their subjects not as the practice itself nor as the culture in which it occurs but as the community of practitioners.[3] Does this cultural community have the right to exist? This framing promotes ethnographic consideration, without overgeneralization about such variables as practitioners' values, the pressures they face and produce both for and against certain practices, and the patterns of decision making and behavior across various sectors of community, be it a local age set of women or the complex and malleable pan-Arab community. In other words, both the community and the individuals who make it up are made explicit and desimplified. Using their ethnographic approach demands that we see a variety of actors and view them in their full context.

This brings us to the workings of communalism as a cultural force. By definition, communalist events are those for which there are social correlates of the practice that make its continuation meaningful beyond any single individual. Gruenbaum has argued that one of the greatest of these social correlates for FC is honor, which particularly in the Sudan, where Gruenbaum has worked, is about family honor and its vulnerability to the behavior, or perceived behaviors, of its members: "Maintaining honor and decency is not merely a personal responsibility in Muslim societies but is usually understood to be based on the behavior of members of one's family as well as oneself. . . . Social customs such as veiling, chaperoning, seclusion/segregation, and male authority to grant or withhold permission for the activities of female kin—customs that vary dramatically in their practice from one culture or community to another—can all be understood as means for maintaining the honor of the family" (Gruenbaum 2001, 77–78). Gruenbaum calls this group obligation to honor and decency a "Shared Responsibility for Morality." The communalist agenda of this case is clear—the right of a community to establish its own norms of morality and to enforce them among its members. But there is sweeping attention to individualism here too—just as in Spiro's kibbutz, where individual liberty and self-realization are so revered. The work of Ahmadu and others helps accentuate these issues of agency, choice, and gender identity (or gender performance) that are involved in the practice of FC. Its practice exists only where there is a corresponding communal support for individual investment in it—through individual and family honor, economic self- (and family-)preservation, and other cultural and religious features. Thus, communalism is shown to be not just investment in and priority of the group over individuals; it is necessarily balanced with individualism, which is nurtured, shaped, and harnessed in culturally distinctive ways.

Ideas of honor are high ideals in any society. By focusing on the broad and historical pattern of FC without attention to local context-specific issues like honor and morality, we risk not only overgeneralizing the practice, as Gruenbaum warns, but ignoring the constellation of issues that work together to generate "good" individuals for any society.[4] For example, Gruenbaum takes issue with the

> spare and simple explanation that female circumcision is an intentional (or subconscious) patriarchal action whose goal or consequence is the oppression of women. . . . This is an appealing argument that seems accurately to reflect both the latent functions (effects) and the correlates of the practice: indeed, in societies where it is practiced women are subordinated and males wield greater social power. . . . . [But] patriarchy does not hold up well as a sufficient *causal* explanation, particularly because pervasive patriarchal social institutions exist widely, far beyond circumcising societies. (Gruenbaum 2001, 40, emphasis added)

Instead, FC is a deeply social practice with tendrils in a variety of shared values, beliefs, and needs.[5] Ethnographic work that is detailed, local, and respectful of difference has the potential to highlight the shared character of this practice within each group and can pay attention to the values that are placed on community and individuals by various moral actors. By invoking a value (it might be honor or faith or purity) that can reasonably be claimed both by an individual and by the community, FC binds each to the other:

> While individual believers in Islam are clearly expected, as individuals, to obey God, the idea that they should be on their own without the assistance of a community is alien. It is up to the community to provide the conditions that help the individual conform to God's will. Neglecting that responsibility is itself a violation of God's expectations of the righteous. Muslims would generally accept the idea that they bear some duty to help others fulfill their moral obligations, even if that means restricting their own freedom or those of their family members. (Gruenbaum 2001, 81–82)

For some practitioners of FC, infibulations serves "precisely this function"; it is a community practice intended to help its individual members obey God through embodied memory of important priorities (Gruenbaum 2001, 82).[6]

What I suggest makes FC such a challenging moral dilemma is not the physicality of the act or even the gender inequities that are often involved; it is the direct confrontation of the communal right of influence over a particular type of individual (a minor) whose protection is itself a moral (and legal) obligation of both parents and communities. By viewing the practitioners of this communal practice as having hybridity and choice, one can approach information sharing and the consideration of alternatives in respectful, nondominating ways. Hybridity allows the practitioners to consider changes that are reasonable and fitting within their larger moral and economic context. Hybridity is also at work among outsiders who respect communal rights and self-determination while *also* asserting a need to address individual human rights. In recognizing the *blended* importance of communalism and individualism, the parallel collective *and* individual rights might be protected.

The case of FC is additionally problematic because of the multiple moral actors in the case of FC: the girl, her parents, her community, the professional/surgeon, and others. All of these actors are impelled by different moral obligations and priorities. They create a cacophony of highly invested moral voices, speaking not just to any individual case but to the meaning and influence of every single case on the social system as a whole. This plurality alone makes resolution of the FC debates extremely difficult.

As a final thought, consider how the shift in discourse from the "morality" of FC to the "rights" of a child, her parents, or a community of practitioners avoids the burden of moral reasoning and attempts to resolve the difficulty through institutionalized rules, laws, or codes.[7] That shift is often justified on individualistic grounds. But it simultaneously alters or simply weakens communalist agendas. While the outcome may be the same, the ethnographic lessons of this book suggest that for individuals to retain rights of choice and hybridity—that is, of participating in the cultural group of their choice—then hybridity itself must be protected. It is for this reason that greater scientific, artistic, and legal attention to communalism is given. The right to participate in the collectivity of one's heritage must also be understood, valued, and protected.

This case is an extreme test of one's commitment to communal self-determination. No such extreme exists at Gila River, but there are analogies in the notion of a blended communal-and-individual self across Indigenous peoples. If Indigenous peoples are to retain their access to a self-determined future, then we must learn the hard lessons of these challenging extreme cases of communalism. In the global debates over individual and communal rights, the human capacities for communal hybridity and individual choice may be redemptive.

INDIVIDUAL/COMMUNAL CONFLICT AT GILA RIVER

There is certainly no correlate to FC on the Gila River Indian Reservation, nothing so physically remarkable. If there is anything at Gila River that has the potential to pit individual against community, it may be the option of living off the rez. For many (but not all) Indians, rez life is at the heart of indigeneity (Treuer 2012). Even for those who do not live on the reservation, many of the events, heritage, sacred places, and relationships key to their Indian identity may be on or part of the reservation. Working as I sometimes do with urban Indians, the urban tribal center (and area dances and powwows) offers a nearby gathering place to sustain tribal relations and identity. I would not be so foolish as to suggest reservation residence should be a litmus test for Indian identity, but it is a large enough part of the Pima experience to put a regular demand on members' hybridity.

Michael talked with me about certain challenges he faced as a Pima with higher levels of education. Leaving the reservation every day for high school when so many of the Pima his age were hanging out at home was a difficult choice for a teenager. Faced with the same insecurities, questions, and challenges of all teens, reservation Indians who want to go to high school often must leave everything familiar to become reluctant ambassadors and representatives in a culturally foreign world. Michael describes how "fast" the white kids were—they were faster in answering teachers' questions, faster not just in learning the material but in knowing how to sign up for things and get forms turned in and knowing who to talk to when problems came up. Despite being in the top half of his class, and being especially good at creative writing, Michael had to miss a junior year field trip to a local museum and newspaper office because he didn't get his permission form signed by the correct person. During his senior year he missed the normal semester exam days because of illness and nearly didn't pass his classes because the permissions process and scheduling of makeup tests were nearly impossible for Michael and his aunt to negotiate. "Part of it was me being stupid, but part of it was my aunt being way too busy with her own work, me not having a ride home other than the bus, and part was just the rude attitude of a couple of teachers, who seemed to have decided I wasn't sick but just skipping."

Whether or not Michael's impression of judgmental teachers was accurate or not doesn't really matter. Factual or not, the sensation of being judged and unsupported, of being an unwanted Indian in a white man's world, is a standard experience for many Native Americans off reservation. Dillan, a twenty-eight-year-old housekeeper at one of the casinos, said he tried living off reservation because of the better job opportunities. He had lived in Scottsdale for a while when he was younger. So when he got a job off rez, he thought he would try to live closer to work and have a place of his own, but "I didn't really like it. You get discriminated a lot. Everything's a lot closer; you can get to it faster. [But] you're discriminated against and you don't really feel comfortable. I feel comfortable living with my own people on the same reservation I belong to, instead of living in a white man's world."

When I last spoke to him, Michael had finished a bachelor's degree at a local university, was married to a woman he met on the reservation, and had lived there when their child was born. Michael had a pretty clear view of the differences between reservation Indians and urban Indians, as they are sometimes called, though the distinctions are not always so clear. He said urban Indians are "more exposed. Like most of these [reservation] kids, junior high age, 50 percent of them drop out next year [in ninth grade]. That's a given. Only because they've never been around white people. You take them out of here, being comfortable and they're being pampered here. Take them up there [to the public school north of the reservation], nobody's gonna pamper you. Who's gonna care about you?"

Indians who have moved to Gila River from other reservations go through a similar transition. Arnold, who moved here from his home community in Oklahoma, where Indians are much more integrated with other ethnic groups from a young age, was particularly surprised. He described how a large reservation can help a community feel strong and protected, but their lack of exposure to the "outside" really leaves them at a disadvantage if they ever have to interact. And this is exactly the disadvantage that teenagers feel when they go to school off reservation:

> I think the ones that live on the Rez are—I don't want to say "closed off" but they—let's see how to put it. Because I noticed a difference when I moved here from Oklahoma. In Oklahoma, I went to public school and was used to being around whites and blacks or Mexicans, Asians. When I got out here, everybody was just used to being around Indians. And when we went to City High School, I saw the differences. The Indians here were kind of, I don't know,

talkin' smack to the white kids and black kids. Just saying goofy stuff. And it wasn't because they were being buttheads. It was because they weren't used to being around them.

American Indian scholars have written about these issues as "living between two worlds," which can be a useful metaphor for those stark contrasts. But Indians have to code-shift between these worlds in ways that allow them to feel psychologically and culturally whole. Indians like Michael and Arnold have made sense of their place in these different worlds by fostering individuality and individualism within a larger native community centeredness. They simultaneously build up individual skills, strengths, and goals without relinquishing their overarching communal and Indian identity. For reservation Indians, this communal identity is part and parcel of the relational life on the reservation. For urban Indians, it may take other forms that prioritize their Indianness, pan-Indianism, or community specifically. These would not be options if humans could not exercise their capacity for hybridity.

THEORIES OF HYBRIDITY AND DIVISIBILITY

Most men are individuals no longer so far as their business, its activities, or its moralities are concerned. They are not units but fractions.
—Charles Dickens, *Great Expectations*

A world obsessed with ones and the multiplications and divisions of ones creates problems for the conceptualization of relationships.
—Marilyn Strathern, *Partial Connections*

In the midst of considering how persons can by hybrid between two value systems, individualism and communalism, I pause here to review a few classic texts on this theme. There is a wealth of evidence—both ethnographic and historical—illustrating cultural contexts in which the individual person, while important, is nevertheless incomplete, not fully human, outside of his or her role in the group. This evidence affirms that humans in a variety of cultures make decisions, act, and prioritize values of both individualism and communalism, selfishness and altruism, isolation and relations. And while actions at either pole certainly occur, and even cultural groups can be characterized as generally more or less individualistic or communalistic, it is more accurate to say that decisions are a hybrid arrangement, balancing the need for social connection with one's individual and selfish goals and desires.

How, then, is this hybridity maintained? Chapter 1 introduced communalism in practice, what it looks like, how it might be demonstrated by particular actors. Chapter 2 looked more closely at the individual, enculturated actor who becomes a good individual by inhabiting her role as a community member. This chapters asks how an individual holds two contradictory values in mind simultaneously and accepts them both. This actor, an individual in community with others (Newman 2006), has been theorized as the divisible person (Strathern 1988, 2004, 2005).

The divisible person is one whose identity is so bound up in her social context that she can be conceptualized as multiple, containing multiple (divisible) parts for engaging in the world. In other words, a divisible person is a type of communalist individual, a person whose social connections and context are bound up in their sense of themselves. Divisibility is another way of understanding persons in a communalist context and suggests that individuals have the ability to share themselves with or blend themselves into others—metaphorically—through their relations. I have found Strathern's term helpful for imagining the moral decisions of individuals in community, regularly balancing their commitment to others with their more selfish desires.

Divisibility complicates the story of individualism *versus* communalism by suggesting how these values compete with and complement each other inside each person. In classical texts from anthropology, the divisible person appears exotic (to Western individualist readers). But with a better understanding of the divisible person and of our hybridity for both individualism and communalism, ethnographers would be better equipped to see this divisibility wherever it appears. To insist that societies are either one or the other or that individuals make decisions following one value system or the other is, as LiPuma says, simply our construction of the Other in our opposite image (1998). It oversimplifies the diversity of cultural phenomena as well as the decision making and experiences of society's agented members.

Anthropological texts about the divisible person represent some of the classics in our field: deeply descriptive analyses of individuals embedded in community context, particularly in nonindustrial, smaller scale sites where cooperation and group reference are so important. In some of these texts, the dual individual and relational forces of human experience are explained not so much as choices or values (the language I have used thus far) but as something central to personhood itself. Recall, for example, Mauss's masked person, embodying his social roles via the mask. Here is a passage from Mauss's explanation of this personhood, as evidenced in Zuni naming practices:

> "The names of childhood" and particularly the "verity names or titles" include not only the totem itself, but its parts or attributes and subdivided in a six-fold manner, etc. Like other systems of kinship terms, these names help as "devices for determining relative rank or authority as signified by relative age, as elder or younger, of the person addressed or spoken of by the term of relationship. . . . So that it is quite impossible for a Zuni speaking to another to say simply brother; it is always necessary to say elder brother or younger

brother, by which the speaker himself affirms his relative age or rank." (Mauss [1938] 1985in Carrithers, Collins, and Lukes 1985, 4–5)

This Zuni naming convention is not unlike the use of surnames in medieval Europe to indicate a person's occupation or place of origin. As this practice became normalized, an individual's heritage and its corresponding associations and reputation were linguistically and categorically linked to the person. It is interesting to study the relational priorities (for example, taking the surname of one parent's lineage, not the other's; having one gender named as head of all households, never the other) that are expressed through the naming practices in various cultures (e.g., Roth 2002). The person stands for and represents that larger group. She is not an isolated individual but one part of a corporate entity. This is the metonymy that Mauss witnessed among the Zuni and could be said to occur in varying degrees around the world.

Our very sense of ourselves *as* individuals may seem like a human universal, a biological truth. I neither argue this point nor attempt an ontology of the individual person or self. But accepting that individual humans have self-awareness, it cannot be presumed that this selfhood is the same across cultures. In particular, do any values exist within that selfhood, or are values something added, something discerned and measured through experience and context? Mauss is credited with suggesting that a different historical selfhood—one not only more communal and corporate but also more divisible than we perceive ourselves to be today—is not so far behind us. This is also the question of our own conversation: is communalism not present in all humans, in some more robust and in others more atrophied? Over time, Mauss's argument has inspired deep inquiries into the cultural and historical contexts of the person and the communalist or individualist value systems in which those persons were formed. One of these is Louis Dumont's *Homo Hierarchicus* (1980), an early and oft-cited theory of personhood that contrasts the Indian sense of identity with Western individualism.[8] He perceived Indian identity in the caste system to be subservient to family and social relations, to be distinctively about hierarchy within a system of im/ purity. Citing Bougle, he described the caste system as composed of hereditary groups distinguished in three ways: (1) in the status hierarchy, (2) in detailed rules for ensuring separation of groups, and (3) in a firm division of labor interdependent with status rules.

> The three "principles" rest on one fundamental conception and are reducible to a single true principle, namely the opposition of the pure and the impure. This opposition underlies hierarchy, which is the superiority of the pure to the impure, underlies separation because the pure and the impure must be kept separate, and underlies the division of labour because pure and impure occupations must likewise be kept separate. *The whole is founded on the necessary and hierarchical coexistence of the two opposites.* (1980, 43, emphasis original)

Dumont emphasized the fundamental idea of hierarchy to Indian caste (and caste globally) as well as an orientation to the whole. This formulation itself asserts a communalist interpretation of the ethnographic data, recognizing not only a societal impetus expressed through religious ideals of purity but an organization of labor and an elaborated system of rules for sustaining that society into the future.

On the other hand, McKim Marriott's approach to Indian personhood was to emphasize relationality in the determination of one's purity, a phenomenological approach that focused on the boundedness and composition of Indian Hindu. For Marriott, the Indian's particular nature was the result as well as the cause of his particular actions (Kapferer 1976). This dividual person appeared (could be understood) through his patterns of engagement: how the individual and society engaged or articulated with each other (Marriott 1976). One's membership in society was determined by and reflective of one's purity, in the current and previous lifetimes.

Marriott's bodily focused explanation of divisibility conjures images of permeable boundaries, infection, and the blending of individuals through social interaction. Dumont's pushes our attention toward the system as a whole, to consider the function and semiotics of hierarchy more generally, particularly as these would appear in religion, labor roles, and quotidian rules for everyday living. But both perspectives—Dumont's on caste and Marriott's on purity—affirm that actors and their actions are not easily separable. Cleanliness and purity of action directly impact a person's composition, which in turn is transmissible to others infectiously through association or action, and (finally) that the group with which one is identified is both reflective of the individual purity of its members but also constitutive of a purity status for its individual members. Through the substances of filth and purity—as they embody persons, blood, food, etc.—individuals become inseparable from the "outside" world. The person is not only formed by but homologous with her relations to the world around her.

Then, an important shift comes in the work of Marilyn Strathern. Her perspective offers a third example of the divisible form, witnessed in the hybrid person of Melanesia (1988). It is a phenomenological perspective more like Marriott's than the structuralist one of Dumont, but the same antagonism of collectivity and individual subject is present:

> Society and individual are an intriguing pair of terms because they invite us
> to imagine that sociality is a question of collectivity, that it is generalizing
> because collective life is intrinsically plural in character. . . . While it will be
> useful to retain the concept of sociality to refer to the creating and maintaining of relationships, for contextualizing Melanesians' views we shall require
> a vocabulary that will allow us to talk about sociality in the singular as well

as the plural. Far from being regarded as unique entities, Melanesian persons
are as dividually as they are individually conceived. They contain a generalized sociality within. Indeed, persons are frequently constructed as the plural and composite site of the relationships that produced them. The singular
person can be imagined as a social microcosm. (1988, 12–13).

Strathern's conceptualization differs from the caste-informed views of Marriott
and Dumont by recognizing a dividuality more capable of organic exchange and
mobile relationality. Relationality is emphasized but hierarchy and status are not
so clear. Among Melanesians, for example, "work cannot be measured separately
from relationships" (1988, 160), thus denying one explanatory variable (i.e., the
commodification of labor) so important in Dumont's argument. Strathern's
description of an exchange that defines selfhood in Melanesia (communities in
which bonds of reciprocity are as materially important as in India's caste relations) is an exchange not between roles defined by society (Mauss' personnage)
but between actors whose act of engaging is itself constitutive of, and reflective
of, their persons:[9] "Melanesian social creativity is not predicated upon a hierarchical view of the world of objects created by natural process *upon which* social
relationships are built. Social relations are imagined as a precondition for action,
not simply a result of it" (Strathern 1988, 321). Social relations are both action
and form—not simply the result of a society or culture that explains who may
relate to whom and how (as Mauss described for the Zuni). Strathern viewed
Western notions of culture as something imagined, an idea presented to actors
in a "specific, reified form" (322). But Melanesians "have no name for the origin of what we would regard as cultural constraints on the way people behave,
in that they do not (cannot) *personify* that origin as this or that category of
persons 'making culture.' A person as a cause . . . is only a cause of another
person's acts, and cannot be conceptualized as the cause of convention as such"
(323–324).

For comparison and finally, consider Strathern's formulation of a divisible
person to that of Burridge, an anthropologist who promotes a more dualistic,
either/or analysis: "Though there is little to suggest that Hunter-gatherers were
wholly unable to seize the event, transcend the normative values, and realize
individuality, life's exigencies and the weight of tradition made it a temporary
affair and would-be individuals were returned to the person, their initiative forgotten, perhaps to be rearticulated and forgotten again at a later date" (Burridge
1979, 86). Burridge's argument (like that of Mauss) follows an evolutionary framework, seeing an individualist potential in humans; that is, only the "weight of
tradition" keeps a natural or inherent individuality at bay. Burridge is (also like
Mauss) accentuating an either/or conflict between individualism and communalism. This formulation is a far less flexible character than the one offered by
Strathern, whose relational model recognizes individualism and sociality (and

I am suggesting further, communalism) through the foregrounding of human subjectivity.

Of these four perspectives on divisibility between society and the individual, Strathern's has clearly been most influential to my own work. An organic and malleable attitude toward social engagement produces a conversation about values and moral choice and not about categorical types. In the increasingly mobile and multicultural global community, the organic attitude toward hybridity is simply more useful.

THE COMMUNAL INDIVIDUAL

Doublethink means the power of holding two contradictory beliefs in one's mind simultaneously, and accepting both of them.
—George Orwell, *1984*

I am large, I contain multitudes.
—Walt Whitman, "Song of Myself" (*Leaves of Grass*)

It is a doublethink that we humans maintain between individualism and communalism, this repeating struggle between selfish and communalist agendas. At least that is what contemporary political discourse might have us believe. But this balance is one of the ecological factors in life that is too variable and complex to afford any singular or final solution. It is, I suspect, a principal reason for the diversity of societal forms. Embracing the idea of Orwellian doublethink is, ironically, the best possible solution—one that accepts and engages more deeply in the process of thinking doubly about these two ideals. To understand others, one must understand them not only ethnographically—that is, with attention to the cultural variables that make them who they are—but also humanistically, with a realization that their shared human qualities are something by and through which we can have understanding. Empathy, intersubjectivity, and participant observation are some common and essential methods for achieving this sensitivity.

The case of FC challenges the reader to empathize with a very costly form of communalism and to ask whether and when communalist values hold up against serious challenges. It will be difficult in this chapter to remain nostalgic, if one had up to now, for the communal pressures of smaller societal living. We are now talking about markers of group membership that are clearly harmful. The reader can, however, suspend moral judgment long enough to at least imagine the values that justify these acts and decisions in the minds of its practitioners.[10] Despite its sensational(ized) aspects, FC is built upon values that are easily recognizable with just an introductory ethnographic understanding: honor, purity, family investments in the success of their children, to be valued by one's community, to perform one's gender well or beautifully.

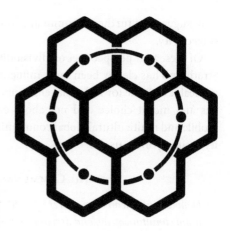

Figure 7. James Wickham's symbol
for the Burning Man concept of
"Communal Effort." Wickham created
this symbol to represent the community values of "creative cooperation
and collaboration" that are encour-
aged at the annual Burning Man event
in the Black Rock Desert, Nevada.
(Courtesy James Wickham)

COMMUNAL EFFORT

A focus on values brings readers to a place of moral engagement and reasoning, giving them a way to consider not just cultural issues and economic circumstances but the moral worlds of practitioners (Kleinman 1976). Gruenbaum's
work (and that of others she reviews) attempts to convey the parallels of human
engagement behind even these most shocking of cultural differences. In particular, what at first appears a violent communalist act *upon* a resistant individual
comes to reveal individual complicity, aspiration, protectiveness, and guardianship in various moral actors. One cannot speak about this communal system
without also recognizing the sincere and deep engagement of individuals within
this system of symbols, relationships, and resources. One might disagree with
FC as a practice, but if the individual is to be respected, then the relationships
and institutions within which that individual lives her life also have to be
recognized.

Communalism is apparent in the rituals and events that represent the group's
history or totality and in the practices that come to symbolically embody a
group's cherished ideals. Individualism is also apparent. It appears in the character traits that a given society nurtures or praises and in the individual acts and
choices that—while they may pose a cost to the individual—serve the community in such important ways that the individual is ultimately rewarded for her
sacrifice. Before the astigmatic eye can see a foreign and unexpected reality, it
needs a clarifying lens. Such a lens would promote visibility of the spectrum

between the polar opposites. The tool would help the viewer deconstruct its binary extremes, first, by complicating its view of space between the poles. Toward this end, I have begun with a fairly iconic and controversial case study. In chapter 5, I turn to some concepts that are less controversial and represent some of social science's best advances on the human balance of individualism and communalism. Theories of hybridity offer a term and conceptual lens to which anthropologists have turned again and again to help bring polarized assumptions into better focus.

Having argued that hybridity is a universal capacity in humans for spanning conceptual poles, I do not mean to imply, as some authors have argued, that hybridity creates internal consistency. I share Nabakov's (2000) skepticism about the effectiveness of any single cultural process (e.g., ritual, value system) for integrating or reintegrating these hybrid/multiple persons into a sense of wholeness with community. It is human nature to remain multiple and hybrid, even in the presence of contradictory beliefs and values. And it is this flexibility for movement between conceptual poles that is adaptive and allows for change. Hybridity is not a character trait that occupies a single space between two poles; it is the capacity for movement around a continuum.

The goal for individuals is to achieve *continuity* as a person in relational engagement throughout life (Garro 1990; Hunt 2000). This idea comes directly from Aristotelian ethics for creating a continuous virtuous self through time. Humans are in a constant state of negotiation between these competing values, a negotiation that is both introspective and interrelational. So a communalist man may occasionally and temporarily abandon his group and engage in highly selfish ways. Life gives us time to move around on the continuum, make what we may later decide were bad choices between opportunities and risks, costs and benefits, selfishness and altruism. Humans can, after all, be successful capitalist industrialists in highly individualistic sociosymbolic contexts but still build Habitat for Humanity houses on weekends, tithe, and pay taxes. The key is the process of negotiation, of deciding where to fall on the continuum for each particular choice: what behavior or moral choice best suits the relationships and factors at hand.

In short, hybridity helps explain how Michael and other off-reservation Indians feel depth of commitment to their community and a complete Pima identity; how some parents of girls facing FC can feel simultaneous grief for their child's suffering and joy for the public celebration and acknowledgment that the child will enjoy; and how Indigenous groups who have been permanently displaced from ancestral territories find ways to relink and rebuild relationality with their ancestors in contemporary practice. Hybridity is the lens through which we can see how the individual pain of tattoos, piercings, or cosmetic surgery is easily forgotten, minimalized, or plainly valorized under the aegis of beauty and expression. Hybridity—and this is a remarkable irony—explains how *group* processes (like cultural definitions of beauty or purity) can be taken on and claimed as staunchly *individualist* choices!

Protecting the Communal Individual

I give the final coda on the idea of hybridity to a blog about online identities. "360 Degree Authenticity" is a platform for considering "authenticity" in areas related to marketing. Blogger Nathalie uses Strathern's idea—that of whole or divisible persons—to discuss what identities tweeters are putting into their online "selves."[11] Twitter, she argues, allows a person to engage with only parts of himself, performing, articulating, or creatively exploring portions of himself, real or imagined. Facebook, on the other hand, demands a more complete and less divided self. "Facebook, Google+ and LinkedIn want *individuals*, not dividuals. Twitter, on the other hand, does not care." Nathalie's interest is in the readiness of the individual for market exploitation and for virtual social engagements. My interest, however, is in appreciating how technology expands a person's capacity for both individuality and communal identification. Perhaps it is worthwhile having a public persona that is divisible, performed, and partial because it serves to protect a less divisible, continuous, and holistic private persona (Orenstein 2010). Hybridity serves, and is served by, this function of division.

In the realms of culture and identity, of belonging and representation, our hybrid capacities give us flexibility to choose from conceptual poles. For individuals living in cultural groups, these choices are innumerable. And it is the protection of autonomous choices, alongside the protection of communal possibilities, that ensures the protection of both human and collective rights.

============

CHAPTER 5

Asserting Communalism

It is not up to us to provide reality, but to invent illusions to what is conceivable.
—Jean-François Lyotard, *The Postmodern Explained*

A prophecy's meaning is not limited to the fulfillment of a set of predicted events but expands into a vision in which people can see that balance has been restored to the world. And where there is vision, there is also hope.
—David Martinez, *Dakota Philosopher*

Normally at this point in a text, following the presentation of all elements in the argument, a discussion of the novel lessons and applications of the author's ideas would be made. The author is asked not just to present findings but to "invent illusions [as] to what is conceivable." But rather than answer the question, "How can Indigenous communalism be promoted in the face of postcolonial threats?," I would like to show how it is already happening.

Below I consider several ways in which the Pima and other Indigenous communities are asserting communalism in the face of dominant society's hyperindividualism. This chapter allows us to consider further the role of non-Indigenous actors and scholars as well, who have responsibilities to build text and representations that further Indigenous legal and moral claims. The evidence of community building I have discussed up to this point affirms not only that Indigenous communities have claims to self-determination and communal rights but that Indigenous communalism need not be overinstitutionalized or dependent on external structures (i.e., systems of law, markets, media) in order to hold together. Having resisted the frames of capitalist markets and individualistic legal frameworks since the colonial era, many native communities have important but still unrecognized lessons for this era of globalism and globalizing governance.

It is hard to believe that in the twenty-first century it still bears repeating, but contemporary Indigenous peoples cannot be pigeonholed into imperial nostalgic images of nonindustrial, poverty-stricken collectives. Some Indigenous people have capitalist, industrialized lifestyles, are wealthy, have been educated in non-Indigenous schools, and have reached positions of power within their own nation if not also their state governments. They represent what any diverse peoples can imagine themselves to be, while their successes suggest new visions for self-determination. Self-determination is an ongoing process that requires a reconceptualization of popular sovereignty and a movement beyond individualistic concepts of rights (Bishara 2017; Kauanui 2017). The survival of Indigenous communities in the face of the agile ("shape-shifting" in Corntassel 2012) ideological colonialism of capitalist marketplaces and dominant global states has required them to overcome not only the tactics of oppression and discipline of colonialism but also the ideologies of control emanating out of the market, media, academic, and legal landscapes of settler societies (e.g., Barker 2009). The community building I have described does not therefore create a litmus test for native peoples, nor does it invite a process by which nonmembers can have a say in a community's membership. Self-determination requires that these political, governmental, and relational decisions belong to the communities themselves and remain vulnerable to and therefore invested in place-specific change into the future.

What is worth recognizing and disseminating as a broader model, however, are the aspects of Indigenous communalism that promote collective resilience and resist hyperindividualism. In this chapter I consider how Indigenous communalism can be better sustained, without resorting to essentialist views of indigeneity or to unrealistic approaches for contemporary global contexts. Specifically, I consider some of the syncretic adjustments advocated by some supporters of FC, the relatively new expectations on the conduct of research within Native American communities, and the survival of communal approaches to healing among the Aja and !Kung. These cases suggest Indigenous alternatives to hyperindividualism—ways to resist individualistic frames (of colonial and postcolonial forms) and to develop arrangements that better reflect Indigenous priorities including communal belonging, generation, representation, and hybridity. The community is treated not as *outside* context to an *individual* issue, but as the *central* issue through which individuals may be valued and addressed. Each case therefore displaces the autonomous individual from positions where Westerners are accustomed to considering only them. In the process I push still further into a deep description of values surrounding community.

CASE 1—COMMUNALISM IN RESEARCH

In the liberal individualist tradition, informed consent to research represents the height of respect for individual autonomy and immortalizes the humanitarian ethic that inspired the Universal Declaration of Human Rights. Stemming from the Nuremberg Trials after World War II, in which some of the horrible lessons of that period were acknowledged and institutionalized, an international standard for the treatment of human beings in research was created. The Nuremberg Code, with its doctrinal respect for individual autonomy, has been lauded as based in a "common morality" applicable to all human subjects of research everywhere. "Individual human knower/actors were the triumphant epistemic agents" of this doctrine (Verran 1998, 239).

There are ten major points under the Nuremberg Code that guide the treatment of human subjects in research. For example, human subjects may consent to involvement in research only if they have been informed of what it will entail, of its harms and benefits, and if they are free to elect whether to become involved. Persons are assumed to be autonomous in their freedom to give consent such that, if properly informed, their signatory affirmation at a dated moment in time can be a perpetually binding commitment (see also chapter 3). In this way, consent—or, indeed, the signature attesting to informed consent—is representational of permanent historical truth. The individual consent process is workable in large part, evidenced by sustained use of the informed consent process now globally. But as a tool of scientific practice, it has very strong acculturative effects and some other conceptual weaknesses vis-à-vis communal rights (Bell 2014; Hanna and Vanclay 2013; Hoeyer and Hogle 2014).

Detailed and authoritatively concise, a research consent form creates a legal protection for both researcher and participant, while it also ensures a legalistic relationship between researcher and participant. This offers essential protections, to be sure. But for many ethnographers—who likely build up a significant amount of trust and rapport before even beginning data collection—a lengthy consent form can move a potential informant into muttering, suspicious diffidence. The result is a weakened relationship and a limited set of ethnographic data.[1]

The informed consent *process* is a conversation between a researcher and a potential research subject, during which specific information about the research is explained and the potential subject allowed to have her questions answered before deciding whether or not to consent to participation. Potential subjects arrive at these conversations in varying states of need, interest, or distress. For example, thousands of healthy college students have participated in various campus research studies out of nothing more than a little curiosity and a need for some spending money. At the other end of the spectrum are candidates dying from an incurable disease who will invest their life savings for a place in an experimental drug study. Thus, in addition to obvious barriers to being "informed"—such as language or educational barriers, or a rushed or poorly translated description of the study—the context in which a person gives consent is not sterile.

So an informed act of consent can be based only on acquiring knowledge of the activity, its risks and benefits. The obligation to inform a potential candidate or patient rests with the person(s) providing the treatment. And consent may be required from an identified patient, patients, or others, depending on the legal, ethical, and moral obligations a given provider of a treatment chooses to obey. While an informed consent process is intended to promote trustworthy, beneficial, and voluntary relationships between researchers and patients/subjects, the process is easily manipulated into a rote, shallow, uninformed, but nevertheless legal document. The quality of the process can be improved, first, through the moral engagement of both providers and patients and, second, through oversight committees, content requirements in the document itself, or more elaborate but rare expansions to the process, such as community involvement or review (Smith-Morris 2007).

Power, need, and access also influence a person's willingness and ability to give consent. The moment of verbally informing a potential subject about the study is typically documented by a corresponding written consent form. If consent to research is given, the form is signed by both parties and becomes legal documentation, or proof, of the informed consent. Informed consent does not allow the participant to change the research design or to control how the data are interpreted, but it may ensure complete or partial confidentiality for the participant and outlines the procedures by which confidentiality would be protected during research and in research data and publications.

In sum, a standard form extols the risks and benefits of the research and its methods, goals, and purpose in detailed, clear, and authoritatively concise language. But this form can be completed in the absence of any rapport between professional and patient, and while its signing may produce some legal meaning, the form itself fails those who can sign their name but not (1) understand the ultimate consequences of, (2) safely question, (3) respectfully challenge, or (4) successfully negotiate an alternative to the document (Smith-Morris 2007).

Christakis lays the problem at the feet of hyperindividualism: "Western societies stress the individualistic nature of a person and put much emphasis on the individual's rights, autonomy, self-determination, and privacy. But this is at variance with the more relational definitions of a person found in many non-Western societies which stress the embeddedness of the individual within society and define a person by means of his relations to others" (1992, 1086). And beyond the exclusive priority of individual autonomy, with its corresponding failure to acknowledge any context or communal issues relevant to the process of research, there is the temporal permanence typically enjoyed by these written agreements. Because research data can have such a long life (through publication and even through the reuse/reinterpretation of data), a community perspective views the consent relationship as eternal. Piquemal (2001) recognizes this when she calls for the negotiation, renegotiation, and final confirmation of an original consent. Through these many windows, informants can reassess their place in the research and the meaning of their participation as the research comes to completion and, even, to publication.

In my own work the informed consent document is fundamental to human subjects research and a presumed aspect of care in any accredited or regulated health care setting. But the presumption of autonomy behind these documents is problematic for native subjects on precisely the issue of communalism. Many native peoples typically have stronger communalist value systems, contributing to a sense that knowledge is owned communally. Writing about research ethics in Indian Country, Wax argued that "kindred traditions instruct that others in the group may suffer if sacred knowledge were to be handled faultily or revealed to the wrong persons; and this would imply that only the community, as a whole, or those instructed to speak for it could grant consent" (Wax 1991, 447).

By this point readers recognize that individualism—and certainly the American version of radical individualism—is not a universal value. Some institutions seem utterly meaningless without it. For example, how can society function without recognizing individual property rights or autonomy? But if we are looking for human universals, it might be more accurate to say that the individual is tolerated, not idolized, across human societies; that our vast and diverse codes of law are to manage, curtail, or control individual selfishness in protection of the group's ultimate survival. The informed consent process is one such legal code that strains to meet its own moral intent.

Native American communities have begun to assert greater review, monitoring, and control over what research occurs inside reservation boundaries or on their community members. In particular, research activities must now receive Tribal Council (or tribal institutional review board [IRB]) approval before they can begin and periodically throughout reach project. Tribes also assert some level of community control over health knowledge when the community as a whole is implicated, as in the case of Pima diabetes.

For research on tribal reservations, there is often now a dual consent process in many native communities—consent at the community level, granted either by a tribal governing body or by an IRB at a tribal hospital, and consent from each individual enrolled in the research (Smith-Morris 2007; Bell 2014; Piquemal 2001). Research rarely proceeds without both forms of consent, but the former process—communal consent—is an important achievement for communalism in a highly individualistic state society. But this communalist process does not apply to all health care interactions for tribal members on reservations. Native American patients, through their participation in the biomedical community and its required individual consent processes, are influenced and assumed to adopt notions of individualism.

The Euro/American version of biomedical health care and research valorizes the individual actor above most other concerns. So this can create substantial stress for researchers bridging between the two systems. According to the principalist approach in bioethics, the autonomy of an individual's decision making is sacrosanct because of a clear emphasis on individual autonomy; and it de-emphasizes the group, family, or collective—ideals that are paramount across Indian Country. Principalism stands in contrast to communitarian ethics or cosmopolitan ethics, both of which are viable—if not preferable—alternatives to the superdiverse (Vertovec 2007, 2013) settings of many U.S. hospitals. Indian Country is one such superdiverse setting and prompts many applied scientists to question the appropriateness of principalism and the centrality of individual autonomy to this ethical paradigm.

Although biomedicine has had a large and steady presence in the Gila River Indian Community, it has not been without challenges. Hrdlicka's early twentieth-century epidemiological profile (1906) gives us some of our earliest literature on the health of this community and the starting point for the nearly continuous tracking that the Indian Health Service, and eventually the National Institute of Diabetes and Digestive and Kidney Diseases (NIDDKD), would perform on this tribe through the twentieth century. By the time I arrived to volunteer at the hospital diabetes program in 1997, the Gila River Pima had been part of longitudinal biomedical research for generations, tracking what was by then the world's highest recorded rate of diabetes in any community.

When I started my work in the late 1990s, I saw mild indications of Gila River's declining tolerance for research and other outside expertise when tribal council members made jokes about their liberal use of "consultants" and some more directed comments questioning the utility of continuous medical research in the community . But their feelings of frustration grew as the ethical grounds on which such long-term, continuous research could be justified had weakened in the eyes of key community members. These sentiments grew over time until, in the early 2000s, the Tribal Council voted to close the National Institutes of Health research unit on the reservation and halt its ongoing medical research.

Adjustments to the consent process for research have far-reaching implications. Repeated through myriad encounters over decades of clinical encounters, the individual-focused conversations that happen around an individual informed consent contribute to larger transformations of community attitudes. Hyperindividualism in health care is normalized, despite tremendous causal influence and implications for successful healing being out in the community. When these hyperindividualist strategies are taken as universally best, authoritative, or applicable, other communal strategies are correspondingly weakened.

As Tribal Councils have grown to require these new processes for communal consent in their reservation, ethicists recognize that "what is ethical?" is changing. Principalist autonomy of individuals is not enough where protection of collective knowledge and identity is a concern. To obtain communal consent, researchers must now address, and negotiate over, a series of questions that might never have been asked by individual participants: What ownership of data will the tribe have, once the research is completed? Will the community be allowed prepublication manuscript review? Will the researchers report the research results throughout the community and be responsive to community input as to how the results are interpreted or shared? (Adler 2005). In other words, the researcher's sole access to research results is called into question. And her freedom to interpret, while respected as a scientific method, is placed back into the context of information flow and who owns knowledge.

Among tribes, secret-sacred and community knowledge is something that, while known by individuals, is a communal property and must be shared only according to the whole community's rules for doing so. Revelation of this knowledge to the wrong people, and certainly broad transmission of such knowledge, could harm others if not the community itself (see Wax 1991).

And it is not only the protection of secret-sacred knowledge that concerns Native American communities. They are concerned also with communal identity and how they are portrayed to a scientific or lay public, control over information about their community, how information might be used to impact their federal status or way of life, and the burden that community members may feel from being researched in this way by "outsiders." Others who might wish to protect community knowledge and identity are the members of a stigmatized community, for whom the actions or infections of a few members may negatively impact the entire community's livelihood. A movement toward communal consent may create additional burden to researchers, but would also help manage the negative consequences that stigma, fear, and isolation that those researched topics sometimes produce. At a minimum, communal consent should be a possibility for communities who are organized and coherent enough to request it. Adding this possibility to IRB deliberations would be a productive and feasible solution.

Among the assumptions produced by this system is a de-emphasis of the group, family, or collective. So this legal framework is categorically problematic for communalist groups (Brugge and Missaghian 2006; Smith-Morris 2004; Sargent and Smith-Morris 2006; Kovach 2015).

As I have described in reference to my first projects at Gila River (Smith-Morris 2006b, 2007) but which applied to work with all native peoples, research data have a long life through publication and even their reuse/reinterpretation. So the community's relational perspective on access to knowledge treats consent as a process, a relational obligation between research and community. Abuse of the relationship can easily lead to nullification of consent.

Many Native American communities have added a Tribal Council–level consent process to all research conducted on a reservation and through which a variety of other restrictions and protections for the community are put in place. Thus, researchers must obtain permission from the Tribal Council first, then seek individual informed consent with each human subject. The individual consent process follows basic protections with international origins in the Nuremburg Code and, subsequently, U.S. federal statutes on protections of individual research subjects. The corresponding international code informing the protection of communal rights to knowledge, or communal research subjects, is relatively nascent.

Tribal approval processes are a necessary starting place but are really just a secondary endorsement of the researcher and her work, based upon a good reputation that emerges from the community. When the relationship or political tides change, an outsider is worth only the constituency of community members who will speak for her. Tribes are quick to recognize and less forgiving than ever of researcher blunders or abuses, as in the fifty-million-dollar lawsuit filed in 2004 by the Havasupai tribe against Arizona State University, the Arizona Board of Regents, and three named professors.[2] On this subject, Duane Champagne urged, "Tribes must reevaluate the structures given to them . . . to be more consistent with traditional religion, heritage, and values" (Champagne and Goldberg 2005, 52).

If both events and relations are to be adequately represented, new structures of lawmaking will have to be imagined. Creating the space—both physical and mental—for communal, noncapitalist relations will be key.

CASE 2—COMMUNALISM AND THE BODY

Heather Howard has argued that there are linkages between biotechnologies used in health care and settler colonial biogovernance, which problematizes the Indigenous body in particular ways and constructs narrow pathways for response to identified disease. From this perspective, Howard illustrates the biosocial and ethical implications of bariatric (gastric banding) surgery for Indigenous people with diabetes. The surgery, she writes, "is positioned as an efficaciously far superior alternative to lifestyle and pharmaceutical therapies, and therefore a logical and moral responsibility and choice for both patients and the clinicians who manage their diabetes" (2018, 821). The "lifestyle" choices of Indigenous peoples, including relational socialities and foodways, are deemed not only inferior but immoral and irresponsible. In this way, two fundamental Indigenous priorities—relationality and traditional foodways—come into direct conflict with "scientific" medical discourse (Smith-Morris 2006b, 2016; Yates-Doerr 2012, 2015). Scientific and medical discourses like these "run directly counter to Indigenous efforts to decolonize health through the reclamation of food practices (Simpson 2017). . . . Diabetes surgery thus emblemizes biomedicine's logic of elimination" (Howard 2019, 10).

Howard's treatment of lap-band surgery for persons with diabetes helps me interrogate contemporary challenges for Indigenous communities. Patterns of obesity and diabetes are products of the colonial and postcolonial experience and in very large part results of political and economic circumstances beyond the impact of native communities. However, where options do exist, Indigenous communities face difficult decisions—and sometimes multigenerational opposition—to change that would indeed improve life for some or all members of the community.

Opposition to change has certainly been present for many communities practicing FC (female genital cutting; see chapter 4). For most of the 1990s and early 2000s, the majority of media—both scholarly and popular—were unapologetically judgmental about the practice and condescending toward those who would choose to engage in it (e.g., Gunning 1991; Hodžić 2016). Since then, more tempered voices and many proponents of FC have established a strong media presence, and the international debates shifted (e.g., Ahmadu 2000, 2017; Ahmadu and Shweder 2009). Confronted with the danger of forcing the practice into hiding, the international anti-FC community reversed some of its earlier positions to respect communal rights, cultural survival, and local forms of decision making. In other words, to allow an independent community of practitioners to change their minds about a long-held practice—to create a new vision in which balance is restored between former and new information—effective solutions will balance respect for both individual and communal rights.

Because authoritative ideologies of medicine are such powerful agents of acculturation, Indigenous peoples are vulnerable both individually (as patients) and collectively (as peoples) to health-related change. I am cautious here to recognize the many positive changes achieved in Western biomedicine over the past century, including antibiotic and antiviral medicines, surgical procedures, pain management, and vaccine technologies. If we also include improvements to public sanitation, water treatment, and vector (e.g., mosquito) control programming, the value of these changes—especially for urban dwellers—is undeniable. But with that scale of success has come an arrogance that blinds some health programmers to the need for locally compatible and sustainable health care. In other words, treating both individual bodies and cultural communities as "patients" demands multiple levels of sensitivity, respect, and understanding.

Again consider the case of FC. Initially, all forms of a range of practices were summarily condemned, along with broad causes including "patriarchy" and even "communalism." This abstract form of discourse shifted away from local, humanitarian engagement with (differently) moral people and toward distanced, neutral(ized), and sanitized rhetoric. In that discursive and ideological strategy, outside authorities were claiming moral—and in this case medical—superiority. It is a rhetorical device with immeasurable force: the invocation of powerful, nonpresent others who stand behind one's cause.

As I explained in chapter 4, Ellen Gruenbaum's framing of the controversial FC debate and her ethnographic treatment of FC in general insist that a community—a community of practitioners—is the focal subject. This use of the ethnographic lens ensures at least a modicum of acceptance for the "right" of those humans to be considered moral agents with a place in the discussion. Hodžić argued, as communalism came to be viewed not as uncivilized tribalism, but as an essential part of community survival, new uses and practices of FC have been envisioned (e.g., Hodzic 2016; Ahmadu 2000, 2017; Ahmadu and Shweder 2009).

Gruenbaum differentiates both perceived or reported reasons for the practice, its latent functions, and correlates of the event.[3] The community of those engaged in these practices is a complex and critical group. Their values, the pressures they face and produce both for and against survival of FC practices, and the patterns of decision making and behavior in which they engage contain significant variability. But FC is a powerful and oft-used example of communalism in health care and one that demands both culturally relative and morally relative consideration.

Chapter 4 include just a few of the cultural, historical, and economic reasons why the community of FC practitioners (itself diverse) might have engaged in this practice for so long and want to see it continued. These agents have expressed to ethnographers, historians, and international interventionists the set of duties and values to which they are obligated. Parents are compelled to raise their daughters in spiritually and culturally appropriate ways. The surgeons are obligated to demonstrate integrity and confidence in the (sometimes sacred) knowledge of this practice and are deeply embedded within a system that values the surgery and honors skillful surgeons. The girl undergoing FC wants to be valued by those who care for her and make up her known world (e.g., her learned ideals of beauty and purity, her desires for her future life, her communalist inclinations), which must certainly be respected as part of her "human rights." As a hybrid person, the girl can be viewed as both individualist—seeking her own autonomy—and communalist—wishing to be part of a community, to be highly valued in her community. Note that both aspects might point toward FC, not away from it.

Because FC is a socially determined health event, it requires a societal approach to action or intervention. In other words, even if some individuals may have the power to opt in or out of this communal expectation, they must still live within that broader community after exercising an autonomous choice. Medicalization of FC has therefore been viewed as the best alternative to an intractable and deeply rooted cultural practice. Authoritative medical discourse can provide some protection against communal stigma associated with nonconformity.

After the 1946 federal law was passed against FC in the Sudan, biomedical doctors were faced with an impossible Hippocratic dilemma: either ignore the continuing, now illegal practices, working only to ameliorate suffering and damage that resulted from them, or develop strategies to alter the practices, producing somewhat less suffering overall (than the alternative) but nevertheless being complicit in the FC culture.

The fact that there are women not brought up in traditions of FC but who choose later in life to undergo this bodily practice teaches us two things. First, widely held autonomy would not eradicate the practice. Peer shaming, a desire to please a husband, personal aesthetics, and some other mechanism of culture contact in which the woman hopes to improve her lot or status through FC are all reasons given by adult women engaged in the FC community. While these decisions may be individual—as in the case of a woman solely motivated to please her husband—the values surrounding the body alteration are not. Husbands' values and tastes, while personal and specific to individuals, are themselves informed by enculturation, institutional ideologies (e.g., religion, biomedicine), and both private and public information. Wives' desires and preferences relating to beauty, while their own, are intimately tied up with societal norms, limits on experimental tolerance, and access to (and valuation of) diversity to which one is exposed. Likewise, the opinions, goals, and tastes of all other actors in society—grandmothers and grandfathers, siblings, godparents, teachers, religious leaders, etc.—have both personal and societal influences that are both innumerable and impossibly complex in their relationships and interrelated influences.

The second thing we learn from adult FC is that the drive to belong to a community and to carry a sense and/or mark of that belonging is both strong and long-lived. FC is part of an interrelated set of values along with things like "marriageability" or "moral worthiness" for a given setting. For some Indigenous groups, living on the reservation or avoiding "white wannabe" behaviors form these markers. And because of the high degree of integration among the different parts of a cultural system, no single element can be shifted or changed easily. Clearly, if the major needs of these girls (e.g., economic, social, spiritual, romantic) could be met in other ways, as access to education and employment changes for example, then FC might not be such a high priority and the communal consensus would shift. Likewise, if the spiritual and relational needs could be maintained in ways other than place-specific communal life, Indigenous peoples would not be so dependent on territory.

In sum, cultural elements that are deeply representative and serve important (especially material) functions in a society—that is, ones that are embedded in multiple societal institutions including marriage and family, economics and making a living, gender roles, religion and spirituality, the process of aging and the life cycle, and so forth—cannot be dislodged without ethnocidal implications. If change must occur, it must happen in self-determined and autonomous ways.

The most successful interventions to impact change among FC practitioners— programs that offer some respect and tolerance for global cultural diversity, and which grapple sincerely with both cultural and moral relativism—are ones that address both the community and the individual patient (Hodžić 2013; Lewis 1995; Shell-Duncan and Hernlund 2000). Our widened attention now addresses several new questions:

- What are the bounds of this community, who is impacted, and who must be involved in any treatment or intervention?
- How do the various actors define the issue, whether it is a problem, and what might be done about it?
- Is there disagreement within the community that affects problem solving, and what is the best way for dealing with continued disagreement?
- Does the "international community" have a "right" that a local community does not have? Is this moral or simply imperial?

For Westerners learning about the FC case, the procedure and its health implications for individual girls and women are shocking and difficult to witness. The community is a source of danger and individuals are being abused. But activists—including in this case both individual human and communal rights activists—are right to be concerned about the larger status system and economic hierarchy that makes uncircumcised women vulnerable (Gruenbaum 2009). The risk of lifelong exclusion must be taken into account when balancing individual and group rights (Gruenbaum 2001). So most activists, on any side, have agreed that forceful or legalistic measures only harm the women they intend to help. Instead, culturally relative interventions focus on education about disadvantages, strategies for respectful propaganda, pledge associations, and conveyance of international disapproval of the custom.

The real question in imagining change or interventions comes down to authority, communal rights, and who is allowed to speak for whom. Identifying representatives, or even representative positions on cultural practices, can be a distorting exercise. Speakers may be challenged on their authority to speak and on their authenticity as a group member. While FC is a somewhat variable event, determined very much by local custom and decision, the debate has now become international, argued by people far removed from these local sites. In the "human rights" moral world, local communities are no longer the holders of their own culture but must respond to influence from an ever greater number of affiliated communities (e.g., regions, religious groups, ethnic groups, nations, continents, genders, the human race) who claim a position in their affairs. A similar contest in authority (to which I return in chapter 6) has evolved between Indigenous peoples and environmental advocates over who is best able to speak for Indigenous territories and who are the best stewards of those lands (Brysk 2000; Hindery 2013; Jentoft, Minde, and Nilsen 2003). While partnerships between Indigenous peoples and environmental advocates have helped both sides advance their causes, these collaborations are far from simple or even universally positive.

CASE 3—COMMUNALISM IN HEALING

If we try to envision a community in the healer role, we are dealing with more of an abstraction than for the two previous cases. We humans have always recognized special individuals with unique gifts, visions, or skills for the healing of sick and broken bodies. But there are lessons to be learned from a heightened sensitivity to what is communal in the healing process. Indeed, much of medical sociology, health economics, and vaccination campaigns already tap this source of healing power.

Healers in the biomedical tradition obsess over individuals, the bounds of their bodies and organs, their isolation in physical quarantine, the sterility of their body's parts, and so on. In most biomedical settings, the autonomy of the individual patient is carefully guarded by several things. Identities are protected and concealed within record management systems, the use of patient information and samples is explained and consented to before treatments begin, and there are administrative and legal penalties for failure to ensure informed patient consent. Patients have the right to make informed decisions about treatments, to have their information treated confidentially, and to make their own decisions about care. Individual autonomy is so fundamental to the legal and ethical framework of biomedical care in the West that its practitioners struggle to recognize, much less involve, the constellation of family (or even other healing modalities) in hospital-based care.

Although biomedicine is an exceptionally powerful healing modality, it can come into conflict with Indigenous and communal ideologies (Smith-Morris 2005). Joe Gone has published a remarkable interview that exposes the misalignment of the local mental health service system (a Western model clinical setting) for one member of the Fort Belknap Indian community in north-central Montana (2007). Using generous quotes from the narrative of his interviewee, Traveling Thunder, Gone shows how mental health problems "are understood to result directly from the Euro-American colonial encounter by which ritual relationships and responsibilities to powerful other-than-human Persons were disrupted" (2007, 295). For Traveling Thunder, the clinic's solution to these problems involves "a subtle form of western cultural proselytization ('brainwashing')" that isolates them further from their own community.

One can also compare many general hospitals in some East Asian cultures, where at least one family member attends and cares for each admitted patient, to an identified patient in most U.S. hospitals, who is usually isolated from their family (e.g., Kleinman 1980; Ohnuki-Tierney 1984). Even visiting hours can be severely restricted. Furthermore, the contextual, historical, and familial details of the individual patient's life are not incorporated into biomedical diagnostics or care, except perhaps in some of the more progressive mental health and rehabilitation programs.

Melvin Konner saw the communal at work in the village-wide healing ceremonies of the !Kung San. In this passage from his personal account of medical school training, Konner is talking about a child who died in his arms during anthropological fieldwork:

> As with many of the !Kung San who are ill, the little boy in question was the object of a healing dance—a community effort in which women sing and clap while men dance themselves into a trance soberly and deliberately—that gives them the supposed power to heal. This ritual, for which I had and have the greatest respect (despite, not because of its mysticism), seemed to me closer to what was needed to heal the wounds of the world—with its emphasis on social support and cohesion and on the infinite interdependency of individual human beings—than any Western medicine than I could imagine. (1987, 10)

Konner, an anthropologist with an established and successful career studying human behavior, decided at the age of thirty-three to go to medical school. He wanted to learn the tools of medicine, even while he was lamenting the contrast between biomedicine's individualist approach and the healing that occurs only in community. Non-Western traditions that engage the whole community simultaneously, in methods so wholly different from the biomedical physician's, reflect a sensibility that is difficult to find in Western cultures.

Sensibility is the word chosen by James Kennell, another anthropologist studying communal sickness and healing, this time in Benin among the Aja (2011). He found that for the Aja, sickness has both an inside and outside nature, relating not only to an individual's life and experience but to her social interactions and the life of community. This Aja ethnomedical concept is reflected in their language relating to health and therapy, in which the verb *se*, used to express various modes of sensory perception and experience, involves an interactive or relational aspect. The Aja term *se veve* captures emotional and physical distress that is both individual and communal, such as the loss of a child or even suffering experienced by families or groups of people. As Kennell explains it, the term *se* in particular points to the social construction of sensing. In other words, it is the social network to whom, and about whom, one is speaking that produces knowledge of the illness.

For Aja healers, *se gbe*, or the reception, taking in, and understanding of speech or communication, is an integral and integrating act. Healers perform their work through both touch and speech because communication itself penetrates, and can address illnesses that are both internal and external. In short, speech is a sense for the Aja and communication a necessity for healing. Similarly for other shamanic traditions, vision and speech are the active externalization of knowledge and power and are often described as sensation that is felt by both sender and receiver (Kennell 2011).

Cultures where biomedicine is dominant largely discount this relational context and sensation-oriented aspect of health (although some "alternative" medicines are the exceptions that prove this rule). Biomedical treatment, focused exclusively on the individual organism, deals only metaphorically with our "sick" society. Rarely are there attempts to measure and harness the "social determinants" of health, although advances in the study of social capital and health are noteworthy exceptions (see below). Western biomedical citizens now think of body parts and organs as alienable entities within a logistical, legal, and separate identity from their hosts (e.g., Nnamuchi 2018; Kierans 2015; Fox 2017). Yet, biomedical practitioners can be barred from looking outward, toward the wider familial, social, religious, and economic contexts for fear of a breach of confidentiality or individual autonomy. Despite their altruistic intentions, the international health community's stance toward native healing systems is one of damning neglect (Anderson et al. 2016), the individualist focus on legal, market, and moral institutions being determinative in the international marketplace for health (e.g., Biehl and Petryna 2013; Petryna, Lakoff, and Kleinman 2006).

But any weaknesses in biomedicine's attention to community or relational factors in health may not be the fault of the science itself. Few challenges to the generally perceived value of individualist science are ever made (Deacon 2013; Rostosky and Travis 1996; Wade and Halligan 2004). Relatively little emphasis is placed on public health, even though these broader patterns (and often chronic negative health influences) have a far greater impact on the overall health of the nation. Science writer Laurie Garrett, who has written two major volumes on the history and impact of the field of public health in the United States, explains, "The concept that individual rights trump the rights of the community—forgetting that these two are inseparable when it comes to infectious disease and (arguably) chronic diseases related to diet, food availability and cost, nutrition information, dietary policy for schools or media control, and the development and mandates for 'healthy neighborhoods'" (Garrett 2003). In short, despite its great successes in surgical and pharmaceutical biotechnologies, the biomedical model of individualized medicine has been costly in comparison to its benefits in longer life expectancy (Stoller 1984).

To be fair, public health and infection control practices like water sanitation, public hygiene quarantine, vaccination, and better nutrition for the masses—while less costly than biomedical interventions—can also be costly in terms of individual freedoms. In extreme cases, individuals considered particularly dangerous to the public health, like Typhoid Mary, are detained and isolated. Mary Mallon spent thirty years of her life incarcerated on North Brother Island for failing to comply with public health and police injunctions against her working as a cook. Why aren't more people like Mary Mallon, refusing to have her gall-bladder removed, to change professions (she was a popular cook), or even to wash her hands (she didn't believe it necessary) when government officials told her to do so? Why do so many of us submit to this type of public control? As I have argued throughout this book, it is often because of the greater benefits of con-formity to the group.

The salutogenic effect of community membership has been a major scientific realization of the past three decades (Smith-Morris 2008, 2017). When the social scientific world embarked on the measurement of community-health link-ages (consider Amit 2002a; Portes 1998; Amit and Rapport 2002), the term "social capital" came to stand for a variety of resources—both material and psychological—that produced better health in individuals and across commu-nities (Smith-Morris 2008; Kawachi, Subramanian, and Kim 2008; Manderson 2010). Social capital is theorized as an attribute of local communities (or net-works) and a dynamic resource,[4] the presence of which is often linked to better measures of health.[5] Although social capital is a theoretically neutral character-istic, there is a large body of research that affirms "social capital is inherently good, that more is better, and that its presence always has a positive effect on a community's welfare" (Durkheim and Simpson [1893] 2013). It is increasingly clear that social capital, not just within but also between communities, regard-less of any perceived social bond or even shared values, is positively correlated with health measures (Woolcock and Narayan 2000, 229).

Community heals. Having and engaging in relationships, feeling a sense of belonging, and participating with one's community in meaningful ways are all healing activities. If we can somehow place greater emphasis on these commu-nal engagements, not at the expense of but alongside individual health measures, we will harness a poorly tapped source of health.

FOSTERING COMMUNALISM

The bulk of this chapter has been spent revealing a world more sensitive and tol-erant of communalism. Such expansions of our interest in this subject should involve a reasonable degree of awareness of the costs and risks of communal-ism. The cost-benefit approach to community of human behavioral ecology (HBE) is helpful here. Where I have seen belonging, generation, representation, and hybridity, HBE looks for benefits, markers, liminality, and sacrifice. For group life to be sustained, HBE reminds us that, first, there must be some clear and obvious goodies tied to membership. These need be truly valuable, either inherently or through some mechanism of encouragement, like being encultur-ated into it since birth. A passing fancy won't create the bonding force that group survival will require. Second, membership in the group must be clear and marked in some way. This could involve branding or some other bodily scarification (more likely when membership is lifelong) or something impermanent (e.g., a type of dress, hairstyle, or accent). When members don't identify themselves in some way to each other, the group becomes mercurial and its influence on member behavior correspondingly weak. Third, the group must occupy a space—geographically, semiotically, or politically—separate from others. This liminality is important since, if one could implicate oneself into said group simply by donning the garb or Sharpieing on a tattoo, then everyone might join. The separation, either physically or mentally and preferably both, ensures the group is not confused with others. And fourth, membership has to involve some difficulty or sacrifice, else everyone would want to join.

Spiro's kibbutz, including some changes to it over time, is a good demonstration of the effectiveness of these rules (Spiro 1958). And for an example of a group that failed to attend these requirements, consider Robert Owen's small, secular, socialist communities established in 1825 in Scotland and America. Owen invited everyone he met to join as members, without severing ties to the outside world and without personal expense. Internal social and economic distinctions developed immediately and leadership was unstable. Both communities dissolved within two years (Sykes 2009, 2012), something a human behavioral ecologist might have predicted.

But the benefits of group life to health, research, and bodies—especially Indigenous ones—are unmistakable. Ample evidence has shown that community membership—social capital—if mobilized in health-promoting ways, is linked to reduced community prevalence of disease (Szreter and Woolcock 2004, 655; Gittell and Vidal 1998; Dubos 2017). Studies have found associations between volunteerism and the risk of cardiovascular disease events and between social capital and obesity rates, even between social bonds and longevity. Although the way we measure "group life" and bondedness remains a topic of robust inquiry, there is little doubt that group life is a factor in human health. Community orientation, even involving some personal sacrifice, is simply better for humans in the long run.

And so communalism is present in all societies. But under the globalizing pressure of hyperindividualism, few seem to grieve a diminishment in communalism and communal rights more than Indigenous peoples. Few have offered such creative alternatives as examples in this chapter suggest. First, Gila River's deep commitment to communal ownership of knowledge has empowered them to embrace radical solutions to their own diabetes epidemic. These opportunities and efforts make them more capable stewards of that communal health problem and more empowered allies of biomedicine and public health in advancing their collective health. Second, advocates of self-determination and communal rights practice a radical inclusivity toward communities practicing FC. They have empowered a vast social network in the healing—and perhaps refinement or prevention—of age-old cutting practices. And third, the !Kung and the Aja demonstrate communal healing in ways barely appreciable to Western culture inhabitants.

If we equip and empower communities to heal, to know and build their healing capacities, and to affirm communal obligations as part of the pursuit of good health—as Indigenous models in this chapter suggest are possible—we would tap not only the strengths of a vibrant public health resource but also the potential healing and disease prevention that only strong communities can produce.

CHAPTER 6

============

Global Indigenous Communalism and Rights

This has been a conversation about two value systems, individualism and communalism, and how they are balanced in Indigenous lifeways. By focusing on communalism, I direct attention to an undergirding process within Indigenous communities. It is my belief that communalism undergirds many other tenets of Indigenous identity, including relational priorities, self-determination, and even site-specific land rights. This does not create an anti-individualist position. Individualism has led to some of the greatest advances in protection of human life and liberty. These include the Universal Declaration of Human Rights (UDHR), the Nuremburg Code and corresponding state laws protecting research subject protections, and a number of international conventions on the rights and protections of individuals. Communalism and collective rights, however, took a bit longer.

Long slandered in the West, caricatured as a failed communist state, the radical and impoverished kibbutz, or simply a tribalist chaos that threatens our global order, collective rights have been viewed with skepticism and caution. These concerns are warranted, as I have discussed, but they were set aside in 1966 when the United Nations ratified the International Covenants on, first, Economic, Social and Cultural Rights, then a few days later, Civil and Political Rights. These address some glaring oversights in the original UDHR by providing for rights that involve group life (for example, the right to take part in cultural life, to use and perpetuate a language, or to participate in a religion or other assembly).[1] By placing value and importance on the group, even (occasionally) to the detriment of an individual, we recognize an indomitable feature of human life on this planet. We also recognize that, as individualism and communalism are not oppositions but complements, their partnership is essential to the full recognition of human rights.

In this concluding chapter, I situate my ethnography of communalism in a larger frame of global Indigenous communalism as a value, an identity, a relational process, and a collective right. The Pima express these values in the highly relational processes of belonging, generation, representation, and hybridity, each of which received separate attention in preceding chapters. These are also ideas at the center of a global Indigenous movement for self-determination and decolonization: globally relevant but locally moral. On this footing, then, I return to my introduction's commentary that Indigenous communalism is relationally focused, distinct from but not incommensurate with other forms of communalism and will require certain protections. I also consider some professional and methodological strategies for better discernment of communalism.

Is There a Global Indigenous Communalism?

The key features of Indigenous communalism that form the skeletal frame of this book—belonging, generation, representation, and hybridity—also build and sustain a cultural group's identity, the *communitas* felt by its members (Coffey and Tsosie 2001) and the emotional engagement with both relations and symbols of culture (Turner 1969). If these very subjective and personal sentiments are ignored, then no sense of **belonging** will flourish and the group cannot cohere. At a basic level, then, there must be a space for (and regularity of) relations among members who can identify one another, who can foster meaningful ties, and who can enact those relationships in material and symbolic ways that contribute to a continuing sense of the tie itself. For such a basic relationality to exist, humans need a common language, shared symbols, and group experience over time (the length of which may directly impact the strength of the ties).[2] For Indigenous peoples, this sense of belonging also rests upon a shared precolonial history and intergenerational relationships with each other and with ancestors and spirits who inhabit particular places. Correspondingly, to respect and protect Indigenous peoples in pursuit of this basic right to a sense of belonging, the global community (including states) must protect those relational spaces, both figurative and geographic.

Generation is not simply about raising Indians but about regenerating strong community bonds over time and across generations. The intergenerational aspect of Indigenous communities worldwide was unrecognized by national and international doctrine prior to 1966 when the two collective rights covenants were ratified by the United Nations. Even then, it took another forty years for Indigenous peoples to be recognized as more than minority ethnic groups (Thompson 1997), maintaining intergenerational, often (but not always) place-based, sovereign communities. To maintain their identity over generations into the future not only will require long-term group commitment and cultural resiliency but must be achieved in ways that allow collective identity itself to change over time. Indigenous groups have had to adapt to colonial and postcolonial oppression by changing certain aspects of their lifeways. So-called inconsistencies like change over time, diversity of opinion within the community, cultural inconsistency, and normative variation from traditional ideals cannot be the privilege of only dominant cultural groups. These are not defects of non-dominant peoples, they are ubiquitous elements of human social life.

As highlighted in my chapter on Dorothy's generation of her family, the dilemmas of reservation joblessness, high school dropout rates, and an unstable local economy are now multigenerational. These may be seen to form pressures against community survival. But other metrics, including the lower levels of commodity marketing and sales on the reservation and the valorization of relational care and visiting (over, say, higher employment levels) reveal vibrant survivance of familism, communalism, and Pima foodways, a resistance to capitalist incorporation and commodity fetishism, and others.

In chapter 3, I discussed another multivalent aspect of Indigenous communalism, **representation**. I used that discussion to introduce Arnold, Dillan, and Virgil, who came together during a group discussion on Pima diabetes. In slightly different ways, each knew and recited for me a version of biomedicine's "thrifty gene hypothesis." They recognized scientific views on their people, but they narrated not a diseased view but a colonized one. Their narratives illustrate the ideological battle of representation and the colonizing of minds that can happen to a people. A variety of English and legal scholars have expanded native rhetorics of resistance, fostering creative alternatives to colonizing structures. They promote an agenda for decolonizing native minds and communities with narratives of survivance, self-determination, and relationality. Globally, Indigenous peoples must battle the representational wars that characterize them for particular purposes. As long as diversity of opinion, cultural inconsistency, and normative variation from traditional ideals are the privilege of only dominant cultural groups, neither human nor communal rights can survive. I have considered not simply the role of government representatives and written expressions that represent a version of history or represent a perspective on Indigenous life but also the body itself as deeply representational in both active and passive, intentional and unintentional ways. In these and other ways, Indigenous peoples are seen to grapple with both genetic and cultural markers of intergenerational identity, recognizing the value of this shared identity while attempting to avoid racialized limits and abuses. Diversity in representation will become only more difficult to manage in the future as local and global Indigenous movements find ways to meet and other forces seek to keep them apart.

And finally, the element of **hybridity** between communalism and individualism is not simply about flexibility in selfish or communal choices. Hybridity allows space to decolonize scholarly and legal attitudes. Where staunch individualism achieves nihilistic and inflexible legal authority, one wonders who and what those unfettered individuals might serve, worship, or value. Polarized thinking about individualism/communalism has led to weak protections of cultural sovereignty and limited creative solutions where communal rights are needed. Polarized thinking and its assumptions also set us up for an inherent incommensurability of types—compartmentalizing both Indigenous and non-Indigenous communities into unnecessary and inaccurate generalizations. It is a false binary. Corntassel names such "compartmentalization" one of the biggest enemies of Indigenous self-determination, separating Indigenous relationships to the natural world (2012, 88) and from each other (Alfred and Corntassel 2005). The delinking of Indigenous individuals from what is inherently their relational and often (although not exclusively) place-based communal identity is a violent act. An appreciation of hybridity would allow greater recognition and respect for self-determined variation without essentializing Indigenous peoples.

PLACE

If, as I have argued, communalism and relational commitment are of key importance to Indigeneity, then understandings of Indigenous relationality will be central to future state-based legal claims. I have already outlined the four processes of communalism in a way I hope maximizes their relevance across global Indigenous communities. I now refocus on one further element of Indigenous lifeways and identity that has lain quietly underneath this discussion all along. It is the element of place.

Increasingly, scholars of Indigenous cultures must be cognizant of (if not also learned in) migration and the global diaspora of Indigenous peoples, usually in response to violence or marginalization, but also sometimes voluntarily (as in Michael's story, chapter 4). As Indigenous peoples are exposed to new technologies and resources, to new media and information sources, and even to local and international institutions, groups aspiring to partner with or challenge them in environmental protection, the patterns of Indigenous communalism are changing.

In response to these complexities, Richard B. Lee suggests differentiating Indigenous peoples inhabiting parts of the world that are now European settler states from those where Indigenous peoples are excluded by "agrarian polities" of unspecified (but non-Indigenous) "great traditions" (2006, 134). To clarify, and using the provocative (pre)history of San and Khoisan peoples in southern Africa, Lee offers several more precise markers of Indigeneity, namely their marked cultural difference including a "way of life" that is small in scale and communally based, with a spirituality and set of noncapitalist values that promote respectful (although not impact-free) relationship with nature, and a "sense of rootedness in place" (2006, 135). Lee's distinction problematizes the timing of subjugation and marginalization in the definition of "Indigeneity," invoking the same historical materialism to which the globe's marginalized minorities also have access. What distinguishes Indigenous peoples from other marginalized minorities, however, is the matter of long-term autonomy in a place prior to that subjugation. These differences were captured in the Permanent Forum on Indigenous Affairs definition with which I began this book, namely historical continuity with precolonial and/or pre-settler societies, and the resolve to maintain and reproduce their ancestral environments and systems as distinctive peoples and communities.[3]

The question of place brings into focus how Indigenous peoples are defined as *either* "blood and soil" natives to a particular territory *or* cultural groups with precolonial ties to a particular territory but whose identity and rights of self-determination existed beyond a specific territorial existence. In the first instance, native claims to precolonial territories under a UN banner of human rights are a threat to powerful nation-states.[4] This argument essentially says that "native peoples have a special cultural and historical tie to their territory and therefore special claims to self-determination within that territory" (Oldham and Frank 2008).[5] But the "blood and soil" argument has also been criticized as "ethnonationalist" and promoting of apartheid in a mobile and multicultural world (Keating 2007). In other words, some Indigenous activists still have the opportunity to emphasize "the primacy of land and materiality" in their struggle. So for them "decolonization is defined by the urgency of land struggle and by the restoration of traditional territories now separated by state borders" (Sium, Desai, and Ritskes 2012, 5). But others do not have a reasonable chance of access to exclusive land ownership. They may be fighting (at best) for their right to free, prior informed consent and consultation (see, e.g., Doyle 2014). For some of these, a land base not only may be fundamental to subsistence but embodies the shared history and space that define the group itself. So Bushmen of the Central Kalahari or the Hadza of northern Tanzania need for communal survival safe access not only to viable hunting grounds but to specific lands. They simply might not survive *as* a community if they are transplanted together to an urban setting.

Still, many move to urban settings. Many choose desegregated and/or urban places in which to live, and they do not emphasize land claims as pivotal in their Indigeneity or in their right to sovereignty (Ramirez 2007; Orange 2018).

The UN Declaration on the Rights of Indigenous Peoples was intended to offer protection for all Indigenous peoples regardless of land base: for those with established and protected ancestral territories, for those whose territories were lost or destroyed through colonial domination, and for those (regardless of territorial continuity) whose future could not be limited to, or even sustainable on, any such territory. In other words, to achieve their human rights, Indigenous peoples require a right to self-determination that is sustainable into the future (Sium, Desai, and Ritskes 2012, v), regardless of their territorial status.

Globally, land rights struggles did not end with the colonial era. If anything, they have become more complex and insidious. The specific political/cultural issues faced by Indigenous communities around the world are as varied as the landscapes they hope to claim and steward. According to journalist Fred Pearce, roughly half of the planet's habitable land could be subject to claims by "customary land users including Indigenous people" (Loure and Nelson 2016). The Pima are one of the few Native American communities who have a reservation within their ancestral territories. The Wiradjuri of New South Wales have won certain small holdings through Native Title claims but lost access to the vast majority of their traditional lands by the middle of the nineteenth century. And although the colonial period of global land grabs was deemed immoral by international accord (and in the creation of the League of Nations in 1920), this was not a moment of reparation, only a moment of ceasefire. Hundreds of Indigenous peoples remain under threat or are experiencing land loss and other trauma.

Environmental activism has variously helped and harmed Indigenous land and sovereignty claims. Loure and Nelson (2016), both active in communal land rights initiatives in Africa, assure us that "there is a growing global consensus on the importance of securing community land rights." They argue that national groups (like the Kenya Land Alliance and the Pastoralist Indigenous NGOs Forum in Tanzania) and even more general, online activist organizations (like Avaaz) help ensure this consensus, and promote communal land rights as "central to development and environmental conservation" (Loure and Nelson 2016; see also Ngoitiko and Nelson 2013).

As environmental activism achieves moderate success in the protection of lands from capitalist exploitation, Indigenous peoples are occasionally ignored in this process. When environmental groups maintain a "vision of wilderness free of human contact" (Bennett 2016), they can endanger not only desperately marginalized peoples but their communities and their cultural forms. These include tribal hunters who, in Botswana, might be interpreted as poachers and shot from government helicopters (Bennett 2016; Vidal 2016); nomadic herders, like the Dukha in Mongolia and the reindeer herding Sami of the Arctic, who have been banned from hunting in their traditional territory, now part of a "protected area" (Gauthier and Pravettoni 2016); and horticulturalists and agriculturalists like the Mapuche of Chile and Argentina, whose battles over land with both government and private corporations have become increasingly desperate (Youkee 2018). In some cases, nothing short of large Indigenous reserves, protected by the state and with no political, economic, or even social contact with the surrounding communities, are necessary and desired by self-determined Indigenous peoples (e.g., Jentoft, Minde, and Nilsen 2003; Hill 2018).

In the United States, a shift in communal land rights began in the early 1970's when Indigenous groups rejected massive corporate resource extraction ventures in favor of plans to develop their own resources, and campaigns were begun to change federal laws that restricted Indigenous rights to develop their own resources (see for example, Sawyer and Gomez 2012; Doyle 2015; Hindery 2013). These developments challenge the "ecological Indian" myth (Krech 1999) and reveal a more realistic, less nostalgic view of the vibrant Indigenous community. Loure and Nelson (2016), both active in communal land rights initiatives in Africa, assure us that "there is a growing global consensus on the importance of securing community land rights" on that continent as well. They argue that national groups (like the Kenya Land Alliance, the Pastoralist Indigenous NGOs Forum in Tanzania) and even more general online activist organizations (like Avaaz) help ensure this consensus and promote communal land rights as "central to development and environmental conservation" (Loure and Nelson 2016; see also Ngoitiko and Nelson 2013). Indigenous peoples are only beginning to learn the ins and outs of resource extraction law and infrastructure, of how to negotiate with multinational corporations and the state on these issues, and of how to best steward their resources in ways compatible with their identity (Sawyer and Gomez 2012). In telling the story of Northern Cheyenne and Crow energy development efforts over the past century, Allison's (2012, 2015) history makes sense of the highly complex ways in which Native American tribes are attempting to retain and exercise tribal sovereignty while engaging in capitalist energy development ventures. He identifies recent agreements (e.g., under the 2005 Indian Tribal Energy Development and Self-Determination Act) that represent "the fullest manifestation yet of Indian self-determination" (Allison 2015, 183). But these partnerships are largely uneven, and as several cases in the Sawyer and Gomez volume make clear, "the act of dwelling in ancestral lands does not ipso facto compel indigenous people to engage in communal, equitable, and sustainable practices" (18).

Finally, because we occupy a hypermobile era, "Indigenous" has come to represent something distinctive, important, and increasingly uncommon. Colloquially, we preserve use of the terms "native" and "Indigenous" to refer to people who have not strayed geographically far from their point of origin since "colonial" or "settlement" eras. Malkki (1992) calls this an "essentialism" that immobilizes natives to their territories in inappropriate ways (see also Raibmon 2005, 2007, 2008). It privileges those communities who have remained geographically stationary since the precolonial era. Clearly, many Indigenous peoples, by virtue of their historical locality, have been violently removed from the very territories that establish their nativeness. Thus, an informed treatment of these postcolonial positionalities must grapple with what John Bowen calls the "temporal element" of rights discourse (2000).[6] Indigenous "place-making" is both geographic and moral, both material and relational (Muehlebach 2001), such that while many Indigenous peoples hope to retain access to ancestral territories, many have adapted to their loss. And critical scholars will treat history not as "a moral success story . . . [but as] a tale of unfolding moral purpose" (Wolf 1982, 5), still bestowing a cloak of righteousness onto current power elites and erasing the heterogeneity and boundary permeability that should be universally available to human societies.[7]

GLOBAL INDIGENOUS COMMUNALISM

If there is a larger purpose behind this treatise on Indigenous communalism, it is to consider the global implications and benefits of protecting these lifeways. In that regard, I refer not only to Indigenous communities around the world, or even to the global Indigenous movement, but also to the role that Indigenous communities might play in and for the global community. Their unique lifeways, including relational priorities, intergenerational sensitivity and commitment, and environmental stewardship, are critical resources in diminishing supply. Indigenous models offer forms of collective power that might inform more equitable nation-state approaches in the future. Among these new forms will be collectivities that attempt to move "beyond individualistic concepts of rights" to "transform the body politic" and imagine new possibilities for political life (Kauanui 2017). I therefore review Indigenous communalism now with an eye toward what it offers as a model for future collectivities.

To nurture a sense of belonging within a community is obviously not unique to Indigenous peoples. What is noteworthy in Indigenous belonging has been the diversity of experiences and of membership rules regarding blood quantum, residence, and participation that make up Indigenous lifeways. How will communalist participation be measured in the future, especially given the dynamics of postcolonial diaspora, landlessness, and urbanization? Significant numbers of Indigenous people either reside exclusively outside of a territorially concentrated Indigenous community or circulate back and forth between their "homelands" and non-Indigenous communities. Urbanization and intermixing with non-Indigenous people are also significant features of Indigenous realities around the globe. "Moreover, territorially concentrated Aboriginal communities are frequently small, resource starved, and (in some cases) weak in governing capacity, factors that increase their level of dependence on non-Indigenous governments" (Murphy 2008, 198). The inclusion of these members in processes of consensus is a reminder of what genuine consent means and the investment necessary to achieve it. Finally, modern technologies, including social media, are already transforming the ways that Indigenous peoples communicate with, organize, and identify themselves. This capacity for local diversity, within a pattern of community that is also global, is cause for appreciation.

Its intergenerational and relational character reaching back to precolonial times, is a defining characteristic of Indigeneity, according to the Permanent Forum on Indigenous Affairs already discussed. It is a relationality that spans ancestral and contemporary social networks. My illustration of this relational approach in chapter 3 described Pima decision making and governance through consensus decision making. Consensus is firmly tied to values of respect for individuals and mutual understanding—principles that for Indigenous peoples are fundamentally spiritual attitudes toward the meaning of life (see esp. Lightfoot 2016, 202).

Consensus decision making also requires certain resources and tolerances by outsiders. Namely, consensus building requires more time than office-based forms of representational governance. To support these spiritual and relational, but time-consuming processes, Indigenous models of communalism may require latitude to act in ways poorly recognized by dominant temporal and religious paradigms. Consensus builders also require resources to engage their community members in meaningful (and accountable) ways. The complex webs of mutual obligation upon which consensus decision making rests must be constantly monitored, balanced, and remembered. These tasks are as varied as the people involved in them, so standardization will not often be desirable or even possible.[8]

Third and with respect to representation, in the post–League of Nations century, Indigenous groups have formed strategic alliances to simultaneously establish a unified global presence and try to redress the erasures of the colonial (and postcolonial) eras. In her introduction to a collection of papers on the global Indigenous rights movement, Hodgson summarized, "Scattered disenfranchised groups have coalesced into a broad-based, transnational social movement as they have recognized the similarities in their historical experiences and structural positions within their respective nation-states" (2002, 1039–1040). It is a collectivity of survivors.

The global Indigenous movement works to resist homogenizing ideologies worldwide—particularly those that challenge the core tenets of Indigenous lifeways addressed here. Their transnational struggles have been described as "acts of solidarity designed to further the particular place-projects of specific Indigenous groupings" (Castree 2004, 152). The international Indigenous rights movement has subsequently made possible the establishment of a more relational definition (or understanding) of "Indigenous" than the essentialist conceptions that were in place before the movement emerged. As a model for both decolonization and equitable collectivities at a global scale, these representations of Indigenous local/global collaborations are powerfully instructive.

Finally, global Indigenous communalism seems to me such a clear model of hybridity because, despite their local and even internal diversities, Indigenous communities remain cohesive and collectively meaningful. Their diversity of communal forms reflects a natural flexibility in human capacity for valuing their social group and finding a personally meaningful place within it. It is perhaps this flexibility that inspires Indigenous peoples to reclaim *cultural* sovereignty in place of the *political* rights that, under the best of circumstances, have been offered to them. For Comanche Wallace Coffee and Yaqui Rebecca Tsosie, "the concept of community has always been central to Indian nations" (Kuczewski 1999, 2009) and cultural sovereignty embedded within the very traditional work of community building (Morgan 2007, 282). It is not simply a political act but a moral one that insists on adequate freedom to pursue a good life. This broader cultural sovereignty is a larger demand.

If, to achieve Indigenous self-determination, Indigenous cultural (i.e., communal and relational) sovereignty must be achieved, then we must consider more carefully what Kuczewski has said about "the capacity for deliberation." This capacity will require all four aspects of communalism, a conceptual (if not also a specific geographic) space in which to be communal. Such a protected space is clearly outlined in several international covenants. As Indigenous groups make strides toward these goals, once again they offer unique guides for greater global equity and tolerance.[9]

FOUNDATIONS IN PLACE

Sensitivity to space and place, the natural resources and heritage of Indigenous peoples, undergirds all other elements of their communalism. I have been cautious to recognize that not all Indigenous peoples have access to their ancestral lands and not all Indigenous peoples have been displaced from them, although their ways of engaging with those lands may have been threatened. It is enough to affirm that Indigenous communalism demands certain supports for managing land and natural resources in ways different from the dominant global, capitalist system. For example, Native American groups have spent casino earnings to privately purchase back some of their ancestral lands. Others use tribal funds from mining leases and tourism to wage lawsuits against neighboring polluters (e.g., Cowan 2018). On the other hand, some Native American and First Nation communities are attempting, in limited and careful ways, to develop the fossil fuels on their territories without explicit naturalist reasons (McIvor 2018). This too is their right.

A relational view of place means that the place (or space) in which a community relates to each other must be large and safe enough for (reasonably) unfettered interaction, must be geographically positioned in a meaningful and accessible way, and must offer enough material value or resources so as to sustain the community not minimally but so that they might flourish, whether in isolation or in relation to neighbors and the world as they deem appropriate. Such space must be available over time, during which members of the community learn how to relate over a lifespan or generations. This space, however, cannot incarcerate Indigenous peoples within their territory or otherwise preclude them from enjoying other collective and individual human rights. The unique additional variable for Indigenous communities is the need for adequate access to (if not also control over) specific, *particular* spaces in which their cultural and relational histories are rooted. Even when these demands require exclusivity of control, they may not necessarily imply exclusivity of access (see, e.g., Castree 2004). Indigenous peoples have, however, been the ones most likely to protect natural resources in balanced coexistence, and for this reason they should be respected models.

COMMUNALISM AND RIGHTS

We now live in an era of "rights," with global organizations declaring these rights through a mix of consensus and republican process. This era began over a century ago. Nation-states dominant in the world when the League of Nations was formed retained their authority over lands they then controlled, while further dispossessions and future colonial grabs were not condoned by the international community. Yet those sovereignties that had been dispossessed prior to that time were simply not recognized. Noel Castree's important review of three theorizations of "space" clarifies several assumptions from the League of Nations era, in which the place-based claims of then-powerful nation-states achieved international stability (Castree 2004, 2008). In the same movement, the sovereignty of Indigenous groups was either extinguished or made "internal" to the imperial or eventual nation-state claiming dominion.

Rich literatures address the distinct sovereignty concerns of non-Western Indigenous groups (Berge 1993; Kingsbury 1998), those in nonindustrialized settings or conditions (e.g., Saugestad 2001), and those whose geographical place identities do not conform easily to currently recognized nation-state borders (Baddour 2018). For Indigenous people in nation-states where the colonists never left (i.e., settler states), the term "native survivance" has been proposed to challenge the ongoing ideological and authoritative assumptions that limit Indigenous internal sovereignty. Such assumptions not only provided justification to colonial imperialism in the first place but continue to undergird settler states' opposition to Indigenous self-determination and sovereignty (e.g., Moreton-Robinson 2015; Powell 2002; Stromberg 2006a). The most persistent of these assumptions is the so-called "divine right" ontology and a "possessive logic of patriarchal white sovereignty" (Moreton-Robinson 2011, 2015; see also Mohanram 1999). This logic gives to the dominating nation-state the power to determine what Indigenous peoples' rights will be but does not question the divine (or any other) right of that sovereign to extinguish the rights of another. Others include legal and procedural frameworks that limit themselves to individual persons, leaving communal processes and benefits underrecognized. Finally, for Indigenous peoples in nation-states that expelled colonial forces, or for which multiple Indigenous and precolonial residents have claims to possession and/or sovereignty, communalism cannot become an excuse for majoritarianism. Clearly, there is no one way of being Indigenous.

To organize this great collectivity, the UN "understanding" of Indigeneity points to several key and distinctive elements: (1) self-identification and belonging; (2) historical continuity; (3) strong links to territory, practices, and economic systems; and (4) the resolve to maintain and reproduce those distinctive ways of life. My model of Indigenous communalism closely follows these elements. Belonging and generation tightly cohere to the United Nations' first two points; representation and hybridity are the capacities and tools that Indigenous people use and need to meet the United Nations' second two points. The right to communal and relational ways of life is currently best assured through the broad principle of self-determination: "a principle concerned with human freedom, and grounded in the idea that peoples should be free to control their own destinies without undue interference" (Scott 1996, 815). But I have written about Indigenous communalism in moral terms since, repeating Mark Kuczewski's (1999, 2009) argument, cultures cannot be protected unless the human capacity for deliberation is itself allowed to flourish.[10] In sum, not only do Indigenous communities require both relational and geographic space to enact their communal rights, they must be allowed the freedom to change over time.

Finally, Indigenous communalism faces the stigma of certain rare and problematic cases when individual rights have been abridged. Extreme forms of communalism can become threatening to individual human rights—an unnecessary and harmful outcome. But rather than deploy these extreme cases in arguments against support for communal processes, we might recognize in these cases the opportunity to embrace the hybrid and creative capacities of all humans, for it is in recognition of this capacity, and not imperialist disregard, that we reach mutually respectful solutions. As in the case of FC, both communal and individualist priorities can often be respected. And where they cannot, mutual respect must be retained; otherwise harmful and violent actions in the name of communal or nationalist rights may continue.

CONCLUSION—REPRESENTING COMMUNALISM

The West has for centuries been such a seat of individualism that even trained scientists and scholars have a blind spot to its cultural construction and to its alternatives and complements. To suggest that Americans are communalistic seems not just wrong but absurd. And yet examples abound of American society holding together through voluntary commitment to an agreed set of communal priorities. How did humans get to the point at which communalism (if not culture itself) is so invisible? For one thing, scale. Simple population size is the number one reason for rising isolation and social disconnectedness. The more strangers we encounter on a daily basis, the more anonymity becomes a familiar and acceptable experience. With anonymity, society loses its ability to self-regulate. More and more of the policing of behavior must then fall to institutionalized strategies (e.g., laws, police, bureaucratic rules, monitoring and enforcement). Verbal conflict resolution, group mediation, shame, and stigma do not disappear entirely—they still occur in the smaller social circles we inhabit (e.g., schools, religious communities, neighborhoods, workplaces). But the larger society now labors under the restrictive and heavy mantle of scale—rules and laws established for normative behavior, a costly and anonymous system of enforcement, and the relative anonymity and isolation of individuals.

The conceptualization of individualism and communalism as starkly opposed is a perspective so ingrained in Western sensibilities that the evidence of hybridity between these two values is rarely given attention. For Indigenous peoples, this is a dangerous oversight. Failure to recognize, respect, and support Indigenous processes of communalism will weaken their claims to and capacity for sovereignty into the future.

Scientific evidence on these value systems fails in at least three categories: first, we oversimplify the way that individualism and communalism influence each other, blending into the specific legal, political, and humanitarian contexts we call "culture"; second, we ignore the moral dilemmas that naturally unfold when these two values are in conflict for our informants, without room for reconciliation and compromise; and third, we delegitimize the process of moral reasoning that resolves such dilemmas, a process that demands assumptions be exposed, cultural (and perhaps moral) relativism be considered, and moral obligations be continuous. Agents in local moral worlds are taught acceptable forms of hybridity and may creatively explore or experiment with others as they face evolving challenges. Sensitized researchers will be most useful when they pay witness to Indigenous choices and relational priorities (e.g., Wolfe 1991).

Social scientists have already dismantled many binaries of the colonial era, including the Self and Other, Pure and Impure, Natural and Civilized, Individualist and Communalist. Yet a quick glance at the mid-twentieth century and before shows how academics bartered in binaries as much as we have subsequently deconstructed them. Binaries may, at times, be an unavoidable tool in the communication of social scientific ideas. In this book, the goal has been to recognize both individual and communal aspects of Indigenous experience simultaneously, as complementary rather than oppositional. Bifurcations do little to explain the subjectivity of value decisions or to expose the intersubjective changes that happen in our culturally fluid, boundary permeable world. The collectivity is an imaginary, in many ways, and the contingency of collective membership may simply be too fluid for further specification within international rights.[11] But as Indigenous scholars have trod this path, they have recognized the centrality of self-determination *as* peoples and not just individual rights or even minority rights, to their survival. My goal for this book has been to initiate more overt attention to the individual and communal together, encapsulating (without resolving) the tensions that create human societies, and to value Indigenous communalism as the central feature of Indigeneity that it is.

Acknowledgments

First thanks go to the hosts who, in this case, have been multiple communities of Indigenous peoples. There are many easier field sites where only individual—and not communal—consent to research is enough, and where only initial—not continuing—review of one's work is made. But among Indigenous groups these are requisite. I remain sincerely grateful for permission to work among you.

I am indebted to Valda Keed and her late husband Ray, whose imprint on me is made clear in the preface. Their influence is rivaled by that of Dr. Gaynor Macdonald, as one of my first teachers and mentors (as I was one of her first students) and whose investment in so many young students must seem poorly repaid much of the time. I am now lucky enough to pay that investment forward to my own students. And I thank Gay for being my first professional mentor. Aggie Coe and Cherie Keed were welcoming and generous with their friendship in the 1980s, and Facebook keeps me in touch with Cherie nowadays. Finally, to friends made in Australia, Deborah Neaves and Gretchen Mahnensmith, my thanks for personal support and encouragement at crucial moments during this journey.

I thank my dear friend Lenora Pratt and her family—especially Deanna, David, Tia, and Fats—for so many generosities, but especially their time and welcome to my own family over the years. For helpful guidance, insights, critical conversation, and general steerage and advice, I also wish to thank various friends and advisors over the years, including Dan Benyshek, Bill Knowler, Mario Molina, Henrietta Pratt, Michelle Blackwater-Leos, Tracy Whitman, Karen Lewis, Pete Jackson, Pamela Johnson, Carol Schurz, and Brenda Robertson. And although their influence has been great, the opinions and arguments in this book, including any errors, are solely my own.

One of the most valuable gifts that academics give to each other is a careful editorial reading of each other's work. For this generosity of time and effort, I have many to thank. First, my thanks to Kim Guinta at Rutgers University Press and to my anonymous reviewers. For the substantial broadening of my perspective on culture and health into virtue ethics and its applications, I thank Tsianina Lomawaima, Dennis Foster, and Robert Howell for their thoughtful comments on portions of the manuscript, and my SMU Dedman College Interdisciplinary Institute faculty colleagues Rhonda Blair, Denise Dupont, John Harper, David Markham, Tom Mayo, Ron Schleifer, Rajani Sudan, and Pia Vogel. For variously inspiring, clarifying, and painful but necessary conversation over various parts and stages of the work, I am sincerely grateful to (again) Dennis Foster and Tom Mayo, as well as John Sadler, Steve Denson, Heather Howard, Nancy Parezo, Christopher Tillquist, Lenore Manderson, Susan Norman, Simon Craddock Lee, Daniel Kanter, and Kacy Hollenback.

To the diligent and industrious students (some now colleagues) who assisted me in aspects or periods of research for this book, I hope the experiences served you half as well as they did me, and I thank you: Julie Kachinski, Jennie Epstein, Shauna Bowers, Samantha Martin, Tonda Raby, Jonathan Barger, Hannah Ashenfelter, Kelli Bassett, and Tim Baltimore-Shelp. My warm gratitude to colleagues in social capital and health research, Jim Walton and Charles Senteio in Dallas, and with the KidneyWise project for the PKDF, Ken Kahtava, Leigh Reynolds, Sean Flaherty, and George Safakis. To mentors and colleagues with ready advice and encouragement along the way: Lenore Manderson, the late Trudy Griffin-Pierce, Vincanne Adams, Jennie Joe, Ellen Gruenbaum, Christopher Tillquist, Liz Cartwright, Sunday Eiselt, Caroline Brettell, and Carolyn Sargent. For relational sustenance in the sometimes austere academic environment, my deepest gratitude to my cohort at the University of Arizona and their indulgent families: Martha Maiers, Helena Rincon, Jen Pylypa, Simone Taubenberger, Bryan Kohl, David Van Sickle, Ajay Wasan, Lolly Merrell, Shannon Sparks, Jen Manthei, Lisa Tiger, Laura Tesler, and all our kids. And finally, life and work at SMU would not be nearly so pleasant without the capable and generous help of Tiffany Powell, Pamela Hogan, Shannon Lunt, Karen Yapp, Ruth Lozano, Elvin Franklin, and Jennifer Sullivan.

Thank you finally to those who give me the relational grounding I describe in this book: Cecelie, Lauren, Dad, C.C., and the rest of my kin—extended, fictive, and ex-in-law.

Notes

PREFACE

1. I had met the Keeds my junior year of college after a semester's study at the University of Sydney. My anthropology professor, Dr. Gaynor Macdonald, who features later in this chapter, made this introduction only after I had committed to staying on in Australia beyond the normal term and had demonstrated a deeper interest in the Wiradjuri of Peak Hill than the single college course for Americans in which I had enrolled. Hardly an unreasonable demand. It was a visit of only a day or two in 1986 but had long-lasting influence.

2. There are a number of inspiring volumes on the role of anthropologists and other researchers attempting advocacy and applied work with Indigenous peoples, several of which are referenced in the pages ahead. *The Politics of Indigeneity*, for example, blends Indigenous and non-Indigenous voices in hard, frank (and sometimes funny) conversation about paths forward—both cooperative and separate—as Indigenous peoples navigate a complex and often hostile path toward self-determination (Venkateswar and Hughes 2011).

3. It was not until the 1970s that laws began to be passed recognizing Aboriginal rights to land as original occupants and granting mechanisms for claims to land. The laws and procedures are different in each of Australia's six states but share several general tenets. First, land, if granted, is freehold, which means that final ownership remains at all times with the Crown. Second, land, if granted, is granted communally, to the community as one body rather than as individuals or to an Aboriginal organization. Other variables that vary by state, claim, and other circumstances include whether the land is alienable or inalienable from the grantee; whether the land can be leased, and by whom; whether the lands acquired include the subsurface estate and the natural resources of those lands; and use, taxes, and exemptions.

4. As to reasonable questions about my authenticity as a speaker on these issues, the answer rests in the quality of my methods and the value (if not also the impact) of my representational account. I do not claim the authenticity of an Indigenous person and cannot offer an emic perspective. I do think it noteworthy that my ethnography was *not* of activists nor of any process explicitly designed to represent Pima community to

outsiders. My data are drawn from the everyday, internal happenings of reservation life. Thus, while those data are less formalized than some other representations, they contain the same strengths and vulnerabilities as any expression or performance. Their authenticity will vary depending on to whom, and for whom, they are perceived to speak. They speak for my own professional and relational assessment.

5. The subsequent era of closer settlements and Aboriginal reserves was not as positive. After gold was discovered in the late 1800s, Peak Hill was established and the area was transformed with mass white resettlement, pastoralism, and cultural pressures.

6. "Mob" is used among Kooris synonymously and often affectionately to refer to "group," much like the term "gang" can be used to refer to one's close friends or to a negative or violent type of group.

7. Long-term ethnographic work and prolific writing on this subject have been done by my mentor, Gaynor Macdonald, and other Australian and Aboriginal authors.

INTRODUCTION

1. See Putnam (2001) as well as some critical applications of Putnam's model, such as Woolcock and Manderson (2009).

2. I do not engage the philosophical literature here, although there are a number of ways in which Indigenous communalism reflects a particular moral order. Karen Sykes suggests that "the ethnography of moral reasoning" is fundamental to anthropological engagement (Sykes 2008); Stromberg 2006a, 2006b; Powell 2002). These topics have been the subject of a great variety of anthropological work, ranging from traditional ethnographies of individuals or communalism to contemporary ethnographies of moral worlds, ethnographic philosophical treatises, psychobiological and behavioral ecological research on ethical behavior, and cognitive anthropology. In short, there has been an explosion of writings on "moral" and "ethical" anthropology since the birth of the "new bioethics" (Kleinman 1999). In many of these, authors are careful to avoid *moralizing*, since ethnographic evidence of adequate detail and context allows serious moral agents to make moral determinations for themselves. Moral anthropologies, many of which take up the feminist ethic of relationality and care, are precisely relevant to communal peoples and may be critical to better understandings of communalism.

3. See www.businessinsider.com/here-are-5-steps-to-making-your-project-fundable -2011-11.

4. See www.un.org/sustainabledevelopment/sustainable-development-goals/.

5. Hofstede is a social psychologist who, like so many classical theorists in anthropology, organizes cultures according to dimensions of interest. Hofstede's were power distance, avoidance of uncertainty, individualism versus collectivism, masculinity, and orientation to time.

6. Rawls's emphasis on justice as the first virtue of social institutions (Kenrick and Lewis 2004; Asch et al. 2004; Asch et al. 2006; Kuper et al. 2003) is apparent here. He names two parts—or phases—to justice. In the first phase, justice is conceptualized as an "original position." That is, when a society forms itself, there must be a "more or less self-sufficient association of persons who in their relations to one another recognize certain rules of conduct as binding and who for the most part act in accordance with them" (Rawls 2009, 4). Justice in this phase demands that "no arbitrary distinctions are made between persons in the assigning of basic rights and duties" (5). And in the second phase, justice is given shape through the reasoned decisions of members within a given society.

7. Despite what I found a useful and broad-minded essay, Kuper comes to a very cynical and destructive conclusion, for which he is vigorously rebuffed in some of the response commentaries (see, e.g., Ramos, Asch and Samson, Dahre among all the comments).

8. See www.un.org/esa/socdev/unpfii/documents/5session_factsheet1.pdf.

9. See, for example, Corntassel (2003), Holm, Pearson, and Chavis (2003), or a number of full-length monographs on the term "peoplehood" and legal entity.

10. Herzfeld suggests that rather than criticize old modes of thought from an imagined position of clarity, we do better to "insist instead on the provisionality of all [our] apparent escapes from ethnocentrism and hegemony" (Herzfeld 1989, 18).

11. David DeJong has published two fascinating and vivid books on the nearly one hundred years of arguing, lobbying, and legal action by Akimel O'odham to regain their legal share of water—one told as a legal and programmatic history, the other as a collection of interviews on Akimel O'odham farms from 1914, in which the very families who had been robbed of their livelihood have a voice (Brown 2002).

12. There is a wealth of archaeological information on this era, but my data are drawn primarily from biographies and autobiographies of O'odham and those who have lived among them for decades or more: Shaw's *A Pima Past* (2016), Dobyns's *The Pima-Maricopa* (1989), Underhill's *The Papapo (Tohono O'odham) and Pima Indians of Arizona* (2000) and *Papago Woman* (1985); and Kozak and Lopez's *Devil Sickness and Devil Songs: Tohono O'odham Poetics* (1999) to name a few.

13. Viewed originally as a mechanism for creating physical distance between natives and non-natives, reservations in both the United States and Australia came to be seen as an opportunity to "civilize" Indigenous people through the work of missionaries and the supervision of a white agent.

14. Two points need to be made here. First, the O'odham—even the farmers—were certainly mobile, as Andrew Darling has discussed (Snead, Erickson, and Darling 2011), so I do not want to overdraw that point. Sedentism may have facilitated long-term, even intergenerational cooperation, but such levels of cooperation can be achieved in other ways. Second, others have examined in detail the impact of O'odham sedentism and their incorporation into a wage economy by the early twentieth century. Within just a few decades, diabetes began to ravage the tribe and has been a growing problem ever since. For discussions of the many factors influencing Pima diabetes, see Smith-Morris (2004, 2006b) and Wiedman (2010, 2012).

15. The results of this work with the Diabetes Education Center as well as the dissertation research in the community that followed are described in *Diabetes among the Pima: Stories of Survival* (2006b).

16. The stark contrast between living in my own little hospital dorm room and living on the sofas of friends in the community was so stark that I have never forgotten it. This is requisite perspective for an anthropologist. Living among the people one claims to study is fundamental to participation observation, no matter what the research topic, and the distinguishing methodology of anthropologists. I have been a stickler about this issue with my own students ever since.

17. The diversity of native response during and since colonization was catalyzed by the 2007 UN adoption of the Declaration on the Rights of Indigenous Peoples and the wide dissemination of that work and analyses of its prelude and effects (DeJong 2011, 2016). I discuss these further in chapter 5.

18. CANZUS refers to Canada, New Zealand, and the United States.

CHAPTER 1 — BELONGING

1. A number of scholars have taken a similar approach, emphasizing the long, often invisible work of "common folk" who labored to ensure Indigenous sovereignty and the day-to-day fight to construct and keep community. One poignant example is Tim Alan Garrison's *Our Cause Will Ultimately Triumph* (Garrison 2014), a volume modeled after John F. Kennedy's *Profiles in Courage*. I have also found the perspectives of Rhoda Halperin's *Practicing Community* (1998) and Jeffrey Cohen's *Cooperation and Community* (1999) very helpful in mapping reasonable theoretical patterns from the seeming chaos of the everyday.

2. On this idea, see Moreton-Robinson (2007, introduction; also see Wendy Brady (2007).

3. See https://indigenousfoundations.arts.ubc.ca/aboriginal_identity__terminology.

4. Dennis Zotigh of the National Museum of the American Indian offers a useful explanation and example of this process at http://blog.nmai.si.edu/main/2011/01/introduction-1st-question-american-indian-or-native-american.html. A glance at the many comments indicates the importance of naming to native peoples.

5. There are quite a few publicly posted videos of Indigenous peoples making their introductions in the manner discussed here, at various events and for different reasons. For a powerful video sample, see https://tribalcollegejournal.org/remembering-standing-rock/.

6. *Mil-gan* is an O'odham phonetic word for American; it is a neutral term for white person, non-Indian.

7. Unless otherwise stated, all names are pseudonyms.

8. Narratives not otherwise cited are amalgamations constructed or semifictionalized from field notes and do not contain actual tribal proceedings. The need to protect both individual and community privacy, holding certain aspects of gathered data confidential, made this format the only ethical option (see Humphreys and Watson 2009 for a discussion of this technique in ethnographic writing). The narrative therefore represents not a composite but an interpreted story about interactions that I have observed. As stated earlier, all names are pseudonyms, and all case details (e.g., details of tribal business) have been fabricated to protect Pima identities and confidential tribal information.

9. *Robert's Rules of Order* is a classic American reference book for parliamentary procedures and meeting management. It specifies conduct for the management of any type of assembly, such as the taking of notes ("minutes"), the ordering and timing of speakers, and the economic management of disagreement, debate, motions, and votes. As the most widely referenced source of its kind (in English), *Robert's Rules* also serves as a symbol of American (if not Western) governance, hierarchy, time management, and communication.

10. Recall this narrative is semifictionalized. There are actually only seven districts on the Gila River Indian Reservation.

11. Johnathan Taee's outstanding ethnography of care in Bhutan led me to this source.

12. Victor Turner recognized both the structured roles and statuses through which people can relate as well as the unstructured but direct, immediate, and total relationality between individuals in mutual understanding and purpose (Cohen 1999, 11–12). The latter *existential communitas* is an inward experience, not necessarily—or not yet—

transformed into structural patterns or systems of social control. It refers instead to the interactional connection known by two or more people committed to a shared goal or idea. All community action has as a requisite sincere human connections upon which more abstract relations can be built or patterned. But the connectedness between two or more "concrete, historical, idiosyncratic individuals" (131) cannot be substituted. Two of the vignettes in this chapter—Being Present and Consensus—address the existential *communitas* or relationality between specific, idiosyncratic individuals. The third case— Introductions—is a more highly ritualized performance of those connections and invokes Turner's *philosophical communitas*, the structural ties holding society together through differentiated, often hierarchical positions.

13. When the world was smaller and the concept of "culture areas" (Wissler 1927) was still a meaningful way to organize the body of data we had about the world's cultures, anthropologists characterized human groups along a continuum from individualistic to collectivistic (Hofstede 2009, 2011). This was a decidedly economic framework that paid attention to subsistence, production, and distribution patterns but neglected the sociopolitical and cultural-psychological dimensions of the social order. Individualist societies were those in which cooperation was minimal if it could be seen at all; collectivist societies were those that pooled resources, giving them to political officers for redistribution according to a culturally prescribed rubric of equity (Gudykunst et al. 1996). Smaller scale helped maximize what looked like homogeneity, cooperation, and rule following to these theorists; but today critical theorists are skeptical that human agency, ingenuity, and self-ishness could ever be controlled without punishment or the threat of it.

14. More psychologically and emotionally oriented ethnographies offer greater detail on the individual experiences and decision making that go into this process. In addition to my section on "Individualism" in the previous chapter, see, for example, Overing and Passes (2002), Kusserow (2004), or Burridge (1979) or autoethnographical works like Treuer (2012) and Ramirez (2007).

15. For further study of these processes of consensus, see Goebel's webpage (www .aboutlistening.com/stories/colville-tribe).

16. I have not adequately addressed the relationship of place and belonging here, though several eloquent and compelling models exist (Moemeka 1998). A sensitive treatment of this subject for the Akimel O'odham would begin with the narratives (e.g., DeJong 2011) and mythologies (Basso 1996; Lovell 1998; Low 2003; Gupta and Ferguson 1997; Rodman 1992) of natives themselves and would consider "place-making" (e.g., Bahr 1993, 2001) something done relationally and communally.

17. Cohen (1999) also summarizes that smaller community size, homogeneity of politics and political control, lower economic investment and competition, and investment in reciprocity maintained by out-migrants have a particularly strong influence on the maintenance of communalist patterns (Muehlebach 2001).

18. Blood quantum rules vary widely: a few tribes require one-half Indian (or tribal) blood quantum, while some require no blood quantum assessment but demand an explicit documentation of tribal lineage. Most tribes fall somewhere in between these two extremes, with some requirement of a blood quantum percentage. Variations exist not only because of the irregularities in colonial experience and timing but also because tribal communities were themselves bounded in new and strategic ways as a response to colonial threat. For a discussion of this history, see Russell Thornton's *American Indian Holocaust and Survival* (1990).

19. See Thompson (1997) on distinguishing Indigenous from minority rights; Donnelly (2013), Sium, Desai, and Ritskes (2012), and Saugestad (2001, 2011) on Indigenous rights in a global context; and Badger (2010) on achieving a better balance between collective and individual rights through submission of tribal membership standards to a neutral, external review, like the Commission on Human Rights of the United Nations.

CHAPTER 2 — GENERATION

1. I did not obtain incarceration statistics specific to Gila River, but the Bureau of Justice Statistics reported for 2015 that incarcerated inmates in tribal jails were held for violent offenses (30 percent), public intoxication (17 percent), domestic violence (13 percent), aggravated or simple assault (10 percent), driving while under the influence of drugs or alcohol (7 percent), a drug law violation (6 percent), burglary (2 percent), or larceny-theft (1 percent) (sum does not reach 100 percent). Approximately 80 percent of inmates are male.

2. I witnessed that only egregious misbehavior, like a drunken rage or the theft of a car or household items, would elicit outright condemnation or complaint. But my limited observations would have been due in part to most community members' reluctance to chastise someone in front of me, a non-Pima.

3. Consider Cruft's discussion of this issue (2005).

4. Much has been written to challenge Aristotle's view on the rationality of nonhuman animals. For a beginner's overview, I suggest *Stanford's Encyclopedia of Philosophy* (https://plato.stanford.edu/entries/cognition-animal/).

5. He drew from ethnographies in seven different settings: New Mexican Pueblo peoples (particularly the Zuni), the Kwakiutl of the American Northwest, Australian Aborigines, Brahmanic and Buddhist Indians, and ancient Chinese. He concludes with an assessment of the Roman "persona" and its legal implications, and its transformation in Christian texts. In every one of these, Mauss found that individuals were never entirely distinct from their community.

6. The value system of individualism is based on the concept of an individual *person*, which itself has a history, although I defer to legal and philosophical texts for explanations of the person and self. Our conversation takes up after questions of personhood are resolved (as much as possible) and remains focused on the priority that society gives to the individual and his or her autonomy.

CHAPTER 3 — REPRESENTATION

1. For a general introduction to the theme of representation, see Hall (1997).

2. There is a broad and powerful literature on Indigenous peoples establishing their own voices in history (e.g., Martinez 2009) and into the future (Cobb and Fowler 2007; Minde 2008; Garrison 2014; de Oliveira 2009). As a non-Indigenous researcher, I cannot contribute to that agenda, and my work may be doomed, as Howard (2003) has lamented, to help "justify the manipulation of Indigenous cultures" (6, citing R. L. Barsh). It is either humanitarianism or arrogance that allows me to believe otherwise.

3. See, e.g., Overing and Passes (2002) and Halperin (1998).

4. See www.senate.gov/artandhistory/history/common/briefing/Expulsion_Censure .htm.

5. See https://nni.arizona.edu/programs-projects/policy-analysis-research/Indigenous -data-sovereignty-and-governance.

CHAPTER 4 — HYBRIDITY

1. Universalism is a contentious area, especially for subjects of morality. Differences erupt, of course, in the distinctive cultural and historical contexts that produce the globe's diversity. It is in this diversity that particular ways of being a "good" person emerge, in places anthropologists have named local moral worlds (Kleinman 1999). When individuals discern their way through the small and great dilemmas of their lives, individualism and communalism are but two of many possible virtues. By suggesting that the work of getting along with others, being a "good" mother / community member / son, or living with proper respect for one's elders and heritage is moral work, we rely on an Enlightenment philosophy of moral commensurability across humanity—that all morally serious persons do, generally, attempt to pursue a "good" life, and that although we may not agree with the moral codes of other groups, we can fathom that those codes make sense to the insiders.

2. I will certainly fail in rendering a complete discussion of this particular debate. Resolving or even contributing to the female circumcision (FC) debate is not my intention per se. Instead, I am trying to give greater voice to the group as influential in all cultural systems, and the FC case provides a pedagogically strong and clear example.

3. Gruenbaum has been an important contributor to debates over FC in the Sudan since the 1970s. Her work has spanned decades in the Sudan and other communities, both large and small. She lived and worked among her informants for months and years at a time, developing that unique depth and type of rapport that leads anthropologists into the most private and intimate details of their subjects' lives. No other methodology, except perhaps personal experience, could capture the complexities of this contentious and millennia-old practice.

4. Gruenbaum exposes the broad pattern of FC across several monotheistic religious traditions as well as the detractors and resistors where we might not expect them: Coptic Christians who circumcise, Islamic theologians who argue that female circumcision is contrary to Islam, and other surprising variations.

5. For example, the broad patterns of "monotheistic religious traditions" are exposed for their patchwork of difference in local and even individual lives: Coptic Christians who circumcise, Islamic theologians who argue that female circumcision is contrary to Islam, and other surprising variations (see Gruenbaum and Schweder 2009).

6. The marking of one's community identity on the body of each individual is an effective strategy for helping people remember its message and its importance on a daily basis (see Boddy 1989). This can be done in relatively painless ways (e.g., naming traditions and linguistic practices of introducing oneself) or in more painful or permanent ways (e.g., FC).

7. When such a shift occurs, it is an example of the "institutionalization of ethics" about which Harris (2001) complains. I discuss this further in chapter 3.

8. See Dumont 1980; and for a useful and quick primer, see http://enfolding.org/kula -bodies-ii-dividuals/, by Phil Hine.

9. See Nabakov 2000 for further consideration of these subjects, including her reasons for rejecting transactional models like Strathern's and for engaging more directly with the subject of the self than was done by Dumont.

10. For a helpful conversation about the role of imagination in the understanding of moral worlds, see Mark Johnson (1994).

11. See https://360da.org/2014/01/26/the-whole-individual-vs-just-part-of-a-dividual-in -social-media-branding/. Nathalie is writing in response to yet another post and comment by Tim Raynor, "Philosophy for Change," https://philosophyforchange.wordpress .com/2012/08/23/the-gift-shift/.

CHAPTER 5 — ASSERTING COMMUNALISM

1. Revisions to the U.S. federal code addressing these obligations (45 CFR Part 46, known colloquially as the "Common Rule") have recently been made that may improve this circumstance (Emanuel 2015).

2. The suit addressed more than four hundred blood samples taken from fifty-two tribal members for use in a diabetes study (1990–1994, a decade prior)—with their consent—that had been subsequently used—without their consent—for studies of inbreeding and schizophrenia and to generate theories about the peopling of North America. It was the cultural anthropologists who learned of and blew the whistle on this breach, although that did not protect them from being named in the lawsuit. The Havasupai sued over the lack of oversight by ASU's Institutional Review Board in violation of federal law.

3. Additional sources (some of which were cited in chapter 2) provide alternative cultural accounts (Horowitz and Jackson 1997), histories of the WHO interventions and political agenda against this practice (Hodžić 2016), counternarrative and debates between practitioners, activists (on both sides), and scholars (Ahmadu 2000; Ahmadu and Shweder 2009), and others.

4. It is variously measured as the investments people make in governmental and civic support, as people's social networks, as the resources enabled by those networks, or as such proxy indicators as trust and collective action. Taken together, all of the relationships, measures of trust, and access to resources are what give individuals or organizations their social capital.

5. The communitarian view of social capital explains that as members of a community share cultural traits and signal cooperatively toward each other, they internalize a set of values and norms that bonds them together. Durkheim called this "value introjection," and it is a fundamental process of culture construction: only through shared values and norms can individuals bond together, forming social capital within and across communities (Putnam 2000; Szreter and Woolcock 2004; Woolcock and Narayan 2000; Portes 1998). More recent attempts to measure sociality, therefore, try to capture the degree to which a community is bonded together through shared values, goals, and norms. Internalization of these norms and values provides a mechanism through which individuals can access resources within their community. Clearly, communalism is essential to this process (Moemeka 1998).

CHAPTER 6 — GLOBAL INDIGENOUS COMMUNALISM AND RIGHTS

1. In other words, Indigenous peoples have had to establish their access to human rights *separately* from those who received recognition in the original 1948 UDHR. As several legal and Indigenous scholars have argued (Bowen 2000, 12), the original UDHR enshrined, through its failure to address all peoples, the hegemonic authority of the nation-state as arbiter of who merits human rights for another fifty-nine years. Not until the new millennium did an understanding of "peoples" as self-determining entities pursuing collective rights and not necessarily aspiring to statehood (e.g., Anghie 2007)

develop. The momentum of this conversation is what fueled the drafting and eventual and difficult passage of the UN Declaration on the Rights of Indigenous Peoples.

2. Note these are precisely the elements of culture targeted by assimilationist pressures of the colonial and current periods.

3. See www.un.org/esa/socdev/unpfii/documents/5session_factsheet1.pdf.

4. Several powerful states (the United States, Australia, New Zealand, and Canada) opposed passage of the declaration in the September 13 vote. These nations objected despite a conciliatory revision to Article 26 that acknowledged the "territorial integrity [and] political unity of sovereign and independent States" within which Indigenous peoples may exist (Hodžić 2009, 348).

5. To address these additional concerns, Bowen proposes a two-stage normative framework that engages both collective rights adhering to minority groups as well as group-differentiated rights based on groups with a history of self-governance "prior to being incorporate into the current political structure under which it is governed" (Bowen 2000, 15). Contemporary philosophical theory rejects the colonial-era presumptions of moral incommensurability of peoples and forms an important intellectual basis upon which the ideas of Manifest Destiny were based.

6. Former law professor and Canadian politician Craig Scott explains generally that the content of human rights within the UN framework is a product of "constant attention" to two questions: the freedom question and the equality question (Corntassel 2008, 116). The freedom question addresses what interests and freedoms should belong to all humans as universally protected values. The equality question addresses who is worthy of recognition as "fully human" (Corntassel 2008, 116).

7. Bowen's formulation gives priority to prior self-governance as key for recognizing both history—without resorting to a "sons of the soil" argument—and communal identity and commitment.

8. Various resources and tool kits are available that help promote these collaborations, including this one by Cultural Survival: www.culturalsurvival.org/resources.

9. Not being a legal anthropologist, I have intentionally sidestepped specific questions of legal governance and sovereignty. See instead, e.g., Kauanui (2017; and articles in that special issue), Howard-Bobiwash(2003), several chapters in de Oliviera (2009), and Doyle (2014).

10. His "communitarian philosophical anthropology" suggests that it is impossible to capture the cultural diversity of human thought in a universal and invariable moral code (e.g., a "common morality"). Instead, a moral world is about having access to a process, namely freedom to deliberate, and not about achieving a particular outcome, design, or moral code.

11. The mirror of culture is a useful image for the childhood imaginary of our essence (Lacan 1968), and the great difficulty with which we can see or touch our own pure, pre-cultural essence. That profoundly and uniquely human entity does not stay still long enough to be captured or conceptualized (Derrida [1963] 2002), which is why ethnographers often insist on thick description of local contexts that may be influencing the cultural subjects we envision.

References

Adler, Rachel H. 2005. "¡Oye compadre! The Chef Needs a Dishwasher: Yucatecan Men in the Dallas Restaurant Economy." *Urban Anthropology* 34 (2–3):217–246.

Ahmadu, Fuambai. 2000. "Rites and Wrongs: An Insider/Outsider Reflects on Power and Excision." In Shell-Duncan and Hernlund, *Female "Circumcision" in Africa*, 283–312.

———. 2017. "Equality, Not Special Protection: Multiculturalism, Feminism, and Female Circumcision in Western Liberal Democracies." In *Universalism without Uniformity: Explorations in Mind and Culture*, edited by Julia L. Cassaniti and Usha Menon, 283–312 University of Chicago Press.

Ahmadu, Fuambai S., and Richard A. Shweder. 2009. "Disputing the Myth of the Sexual Dysfunction of Circumcised Women: An Interview with Fuambai S. Ahmadu by Richard A. Shweder." *Anthropology Today* 25 (6):14–17.

Aknin, Lara B., Christopher P. Barrington-Leigh, Elizabeth W. Dunn, John F. Helliwell, Justine Burns, Robert Biswas-Diener, Imelda Kemeza, Paul Nyende, Claire E. Ashton-James, and Michael I. Norton. 2013. "Prosocial Spending and Well-Being: Cross-Cultural Evidence for a Psychological Universal." *Journal of Personality and Social Psychology* 104 (4):635–652.

Alfred, Taiaiake, and Jeff Corntassel. 2005. "Being Indigenous: Resurgences against Contemporary Colonialism." *Government and Opposition* 40 (4): 597–614.

Allison, James. 2012. "From Survival to Sovereignty: 1970s Energy Development and Indian Self-Determination in Montana's Powder River Basin." *Environmental Justice* 5 (5):252–263.

———. 2015. *Sovereignty for Survival: American Energy Development and Indian Self-Determination.* Yale University Press.

Amit, Vered. 2002a. *Realizing Community: Concepts, Social Relationships and Sentiments.* Psychology Press.

———. 2002b. "Reconceptualizing Community." In Amit, *Realizing Community*, 11–30. Routledge.

Amit, Vered, and Nigel Rapport. 2002. *The Trouble with Community: Anthropological Reflections on Movement, Identity and Collectivity.* Pluto Press.

Anderson, Ian, Bridget Robson, Michele Connolly, Fadwa Al-Yaman, Espen Bjertness, Alexandra King, Michael Tynan, Richard Madden, Abhay Bang, and Carlos E. A. Coimbra Jr. 2016. "Indigenous and Tribal Peoples' Health (The Lancet–Lowitja Institute Global Collaboration): A Population Study." *Lancet* 388 (10040):131–157.

Anderson, Lisa R., Francis J. DiTraglia, and Jeffrey R. Gerlach. 2011. "Measuring Altruism in a Public Goods Experiment: A Comparison of US and Czech Subjects." *Experimental Economics* 14 (3):426–437.

Anderson, Warwick. 2014. "Making Global Health History: The Postcolonial Worldliness of Biomedicine." *Social History of Medicine* 27 (2):372–384.

Andranovich, Greg. 1995. "Achieving Consensus in Public Decision Making: Applying Interest-Based Problem Solving to the Challenges of Intergovernmental Collaboration." *Journal of Applied Behavioral Science* 31 (4):429–445. doi:10.1177/0021886395314003.

Anghie, Antony. 2007. *Imperialism, Sovereignty and the Making of International Law.* Vol. 37. Cambridge University Press.

Annas, George J., and Sherman Elias. 2014. "23andMe and the FDA." *New England Journal of Medicine* 370 (11):985–988.

Asch, Michael, Colin Samson, Ulf Dahre, and Adam Kuper. 2006. "More on the Return of the Native." *Current Anthropology* 47 (1):145–149.

Asch, Michael, Colin Samson, Dieter Heinen, Justin Kenrick, Jerome Lewis, Sidsel Saugestad, Terry Turner, and Adam Kuper. 2004. "On the Return of the Native." *Current Anthropology* 45 (2):261–267.

Ashton, Michael C., and Kibeom Lee. 2007. "Empirical, Theoretical, and Practical Advantages of the HEXACO Model of Personality Structure." *Personality and Social Psychology Review* 11 (2):150–166.

Ayub, Qasim, Loukas Moutsianas, Yuan Chen, Kalliope Panoutsopoulou, Vincenza Colonna, Luca Pagani, Inga Prokopenko, Graham R. S. Ritchie, Chris Tyler-Smith, and Mark I. McCarthy. 2014. "Revisiting the Thrifty Gene Hypothesis via 65 Loci Associated with Susceptibility to Type 2 Diabetes." *American Journal of Human Genetics* 94 (2):176–185.

Baddour, Dylan. 2018. "Not welcome in Colombia, Indigenous Migrants Stuck at Border after Fleeing Venezuela." *The Guardian,* April 23.

Badger, Austin. 2010. "Collective v. Individual Human Rights in Membership Governance for Indigenous Peoples." *American University International Law Review* 26:485–514.

Bahr, Donald. 1993. "What Happened to Mythology?" *Wicazo Sa Review October*:44–49.

———. 2001. "Bad News: The Predicament of Native American Mythology." *Ethnohistory* 48 (4):587–612.

Bahti, Tom. 1968. *Southwestern Indian Tribes.* KC Publications.

Barker, Adam J. 2009. "The Contemporary Reality of Canadian Imperialism: Settler Colonialism and the Hybrid Colonial State." *American Indian Quarterly* 33 (3): 325–351.

Barnard, Alan. 2006. "Kalahari Revisionism, Vienna and the 'Indigenous Peoples' Debate." *Social Anthropology* 14 (1): 1–16.

Basso, Keith H. 1996. "Wisdom Sits in Places: Notes on a Western Apache Landscape." In *Sense of Place,* edited by Steven Feld and Keith H. Basso, 53–90. School of American Research Press.

Bell, Kirsten. 2014. "Resisting Commensurability: Against Informed Consent as an Anthropological Virtue." *American Anthropologist* 116 (3):511–522.

Bennett, Gordon. 2016. "Hunting Must Be Regarded as a Human Right for Indigenous and Tribal Peoples." *The Guardian,* December 16.

Berge, Erling. 1994. "Culture, Property Rights Regimes and Resource Utilization." *Law and the Management of Divisible and Non-Excludable Renewable Resources,* edited by Erling Berge, Derek Ott, and Nils Chr. Stenseth, 3–30. The Agricultural University of Norway.

Bernstein, Mary. 1997. "Celebration and Suppression: The Strategic Uses of Identity by the Lesbian and Gay Movement." *American Journal of Sociology* 103 (3):531–565.

Bhabha, Homi K. 1994. *The Location of Culture.* Routledge.

Biehl, João, and Adriana Petryna. 2013. *When People Come First: Critical Studies in Global Health.* Princeton, NJ: Princeton University Press.

Bishara, Amahl. 2017. "Sovereignty and Popular Sovereignty for Palestinians and Beyond." *Cultural Anthropology* 32 (3):349–358.

Boddy, Janice. 1989. *Wombs and Alien Spirits: Women, Men, and the Zar Cult in Northern Sudan.* University of Wisconsin Press.

Boldt, Menno. 1993. *Surviving as Indians: The Challenge of Self-Government.* University of Toronto Press.

Bowen, John R. 2000. "Should We Have a Universal Concept of 'Indigenous Peoples' Rights'? Ethnicity and Essentialism in the Twenty-First Century." *Anthropology Today* 16 (4):12–16.

Brady, Wendy. 2007. "That Sovereign Being: History Matters." In Moreton-Robinson, *Sovereign Subjects: Indigenous Sovereignty Matters,* 140–152.

Brenneman, Dale S. 2014. "Bringing O'odham into the 'Pimería Alta': Introduction." *Journal of the Southwest* 56 (2): 205–218.

Brown, Cynthia G. 1995. *Playing the" Communal Card": Communal Violence and Human Rights.* Vol. 2156. Human Rights Watch.

Brown, Susan Love. 2002. *Intentional Community: An Anthropological Perspective.* State University of New York Press.

Brugge, Doug, and Mariam Missaghian. 2006. "Protecting the Navajo People through Tribal Regulation of Research." *Science and Engineering Ethics* 12 (3):491–507.

Brysk, Alison. 2000. *From Tribal Village to Global Village: Indian Rights and International Relations in Latin America.* Stanford University Press.

Burridge, Kenelm. 1979. *Someone, No One: An Essay on Individuality.* Princeton University Press.

Cameron, Sue. 2013. "A Barbaric Practice That Shames Us All." *Daily Telegraph,* June 12.

Canby, William, Jr. 2014. *American Indian Law in a Nutshell.* 6th ed. West Academic.

Carrithers, Michael, Steven Collins, and Steven Lukes. 1985. *The Category of the Person: Anthropology, Philosophy, History.* Cambridge University Press.

Castellino, Joshua, and Jérémie Gilbert. 2003. "Self-determination, Indigenous Peoples and Minorities." *Macquarie Law Journal* 3: 155.

Castetter, E.F., and W.H. Bell. 1942. *Pima and Papago Indian Agriculture.* Inter-Americana Studies I. University of New Mexico Press.

Castree, Noel. 2004. "Differential Geographies: Place, Indigenous Rights and 'Local' Resources." *Political Geography* 23 (2):133–167.

———. 2008. "Neoliberalising Nature: Processes, Effects, and Evaluations." *Environment and Planning A* 40 (1):153–173.

Champagne, Duane, and Carole E. Goldberg. 2005. "Changing the Subject: Individual versus Collective Interests in Indian Country Research." *Wicazo Sa Review* 20 (1):49–69.

Christakis, Nicholas A. 1992. "Ethics Are Local: Engaging Cross-Cultural Variation in the Ethics for Clinical Research." *Social Science & Medicine* 35 (9):1079–1091. doi:10.1016/0277-9536(92)90220-K.

Cobb, Daniel M., and Loretta Fowler, eds. 2007. *Beyond Red Power: American Indian Politics and Activism since 1900.* School for Advanced Research Press.

Cochran, Patricia A. L., Catherine A. Marshall, Carmen Garcia-Downing, Elizabeth Kendall, Doris Cook, Laurie McCubbin, and Reva Mariah S. Gover. 2008. "Indigenous Ways of Knowing: Implications for Participatory Research and Community." *American Journal of Public Health* 98 (1):22–27.

Coffey, Wallace, and Rebecca Tsosie. 2001. "Rethinking the Tribal Sovereignty Doctrine: Cultural Sovereignty and the Collective Future of Indian Nations." *Stanford Law and Policy Review* 12:191–222.

Cohen, Jeffrey H. 1999. *Cooperation and Community: Economy and Society in Oaxaca.* Austin: University of Texas Press.

Conklin, Beth A. 2002. "Shamans versus Pirates in the Amazonian Treasure Chest." *American Anthropologist* 104 (4):1050–1061.

Conklin, Beth A., and Laura R. Graham. 1995. "The Shifting Middle Ground: Amazonian Indians and Eco-politics." *American Anthropologist* 97 (4):695–710.

Corntassel, Jeff. 2003. "Who Is Indigenous? 'Peoplehood' and Ethnonationalist Approaches to Rearticulating Indigenous Identity." *Nationalism and Ethnic Politics* 9 (1):75–100.

———. 2008. "Toward Sustainable Self-Determination: Rethinking the Contemporary Indigenous-Rights Discourse." *Alternatives* 33 (1):105–132.

———. 2012. "Re-Envisioning Resurgence: Indigenous Pathways to Decolonization and Sustainable Self-determination." *Decolonization: Indigeneity, Education & Society* 1(1): 86–101.

Cowan, Emery. 2018. "US Tribe Fights Use of Treated Sewage to Make Snow on Holy Peaks." *The Guardian*, February 15.Curry, Oliver, Sam G. B. Roberts, and Robin I. M. Dunbar. 2013. "Altruism in Social Networks: Evidence for a 'Kinship Premium.'" *British Journal of Psychology* 104 (2):283–295.

Darling, J. Andrew, Barnaby V. Lewis, Robert Valencia, and B. Sunday Eiselt. 2015. "Archaeology in the Service of the Tribe: Three Episodes in Twenty-First-Century Tribal Archaeology in the US–Mexico Borderlands." *Kiva* 81 (1–2):62–79.

Deacon, Brett J. 2013. "The Biomedical Model of Mental Disorder: A Critical Analysis of Its Validity, Utility, and Effects on Psychotherapy Research." *Clinical Psychology Review* 33 (7):846–861.

DeJong, David H. 2003. "A SCHEME TO ROB THEM OF THEIR LAND: Water, Allotment, and the Economic Integration of the Pima Reservation, 1902–1921." *The Journal of Arizona History* 44 (2): 99–132.

———. 2011. *Forced to Abandon Our Fields: The 1914 Clay Southworth Gila River Pima Interviews.* University of Utah Press.

———. 2016. *Stealing the Gila: The Pima Agricultural Economy and Water Deprivation, 1848–1921.* University of Arizona Press.

DeLanda, Manuel. 2006. *A New Philosophy of Society: Assemblage Theory and Social Complexity*. Bloomsbury.

de Oliveira, Adolfo, ed. 2009. *Decolonising Indigenous Rights*. Routledge.

Derrida, Jacques. [1963] 2002. "Force and Signification." *J. Derrida, Writing and Difference*. Translated by Alan Bass, 1–35. Routledge.

Diamond, Jared. 1987. "The Worst Mistake in the History of the Human Race." *Discover* 8 (5):64–66.

———. 1997. *Guns, Germs, and Steel: The Fates of Human Societies*. Norton.

Dobyns, Henry F. 1989. *The Pima-Maricopa*. Chelsea House.

Donnelly, Jack. 2013. *Universal Human Rights in Theory and Practice*. Cornell University Press.

Doyle, Cathal M. 2014. *Indigenous Peoples, Title to Territory, Rights and Resources: The Transformative Role of Free Prior and Informed Consent*. Routledge.

Dubos, Rene. 2017. *Social Capital: Theory and Research*. Routledge.

Dumont, Louis. 1980. *Homo Hierarchicus: The Caste System and Its Implications*. University of Chicago Press.

Durkheim, Émile, and George Simpson. [1893] 2013. *The Division of Labor in Society*. Macmillan International Higher Education.

Echo-Hawk, Walter R. 2016. *In the Light of Justice: The Rise of Human Rights in Native America and the UN Declaration on the Rights of Indigenous Peoples*. Fulcrum Publishing.

Emanuel, Ezekiel J. 2015. "Reform of Clinical Research Regulations, Finally." *New England Journal of Medicine* 373 (24):2296–2299.

Etzioni, Amitai. 1998. *The Essential Communitarian Reader*. Rowman & Littlefield.

Fagan, Brian M. 2006. *Ancient North America: The Archaeology of a Continent*. Thames & Hudson.

Farmer, Paul, Philippe Bourgois, Nancy Scheper-Hughes, Didier Fassin, Linda Green, H. K. Heggenhougen, Laurence Kirmayer, and Loc Wacquant. 2004. "An Anthropology of Structural Violence." *Current Anthropology* 45 (3):305–325.

Fletcher, Matthew L. M. 2012. "Tribal Membership and Indian Nationhood." *American Indian Law Review* 37:1–18.

Foner, Nancy. 1997. "The Immigrant Family: Cultural Legacies and Cultural Changes." *International Migration Review* 31 (4):961–974.

———, ed. 2003. *American Arrivals: Anthropology Engages the New Immigration*. School of American Research Press.

Fox, Renée C. 2017. *Spare Parts: Organ Replacement in American Society*. Routledge.

Fry, Peter. 1976. *Spirits of Protest: Spirit-Mediums and the Articulation of Consensus among the Zezuru of Southern Rhodesia (Zimbabwe)*. Cambridge University Press.

Garrett, Laurie. 2003. *Betrayal of Trust: The Collapse of Global Public Health*. Oxford University Press.

Garrison, Tim Alan. 2014. *Our Cause Will Ultimately Triumph: Profiles in American Indian Sovereignty*. Carolina Academic Press.

Garro, Linda C. 1990. "Continuity and Change: The Interpretation of Illness in an Anishinaabe (Ojibway) Community." *Culture, Medicine and Psychiatry* 14 (4):417–454.

Gauthier, Marine, and Riccardo Pravettoni. 2016. "'We Have Nothing but Our Reindeer': Conservation Threatens Ruination for Mongolia's Dukha." *The Guardian*, August 28.

Geertz, Clifford. 1973. *The Interpretation of Cultures*. Basic Books.

Ghiglieri, Michael Patrick, and Thomas M. Myers. 2001. *Over the Edge: Death in Grand Canyon: Gripping Accounts of All Known Fatal Mishaps in the Most Famous of the World's Seven Natural Wonders*. Puma Press.

Gittell, Ross, and Avis Vidal. 1998. *Community Organizing: Building Social Capital as a Development Strategy*. Sage.

Gomez, Lauren. 2016. "Beyond Black and White: Native American Representation in Mainstream Media."Master's thesis, University of Oklahoma. https://hdl.handle.net /11244/34640.

Gone, Joseph P. 2007. ""We Never Was Happy Living Like a Whiteman": Mental Health Disparities and the Postcolonial Predicament in American Indian Communities." *American Journal of Community Psychology* 40 (3–4): 290–300.

Gruenbaum, Ellen. 2001. *The Female Circumcision Controversy: An Anthropological Perspective*. University of Pennsylvania Press.

———. 2009. "Honorable Mutilation? Changing Responses to Female Genital Cutting in Sudan." In *Anthropology and Public Health: Bridging Difference in Culture and Society*, edited by Robert A. Hahn and Marcia Inborn, 397–421. Oxford University Press.

Gudykunst, William B., Yuko Matsumoto, Stella Ting-Toomey, Tsukasa Nishida, Kwangsu Kim, and Sam Heyman. 1996. "The Influence of Cultural Individualism-Collectivism, Self Construals, and Individual Values on Communication Styles across Cultures." *Human Communication Research* 22 (4):510–543.

Guillory, Raphael M., and Mimi Wolverton. 2008. "It's about Family: Native American Student Persistence in Higher Education." *Journal of Higher Education* 79 (1):58–87.

Gunning, Isabelle R. 1991. "Arrogant Perception, World-Travelling and Multicultural Feminism: The Case of Female Genital Surgeries." *Columbia Human Rights Law Review* 23:189–248.

Gupta, Akhil, and James Ferguson. 1997. *Culture, Power, Place: Explorations in Critical Anthropology*. Duke University Press.

Hackenberg, Robert A. 1962. "Economic Alternatives in Arid Lands: A Case Study of the Pima and Papago Indians." *Ethnology* 1 (2): 186–196.

Hale, Charles R. 2006. "Activist Research v. Cultural Critique: Indigenous Land Rights and the Contradictions of Politically Engaged Anthropology." *Cultural Anthropology* 21 (1): 96–120.

Halgunseth, Linda C., Jean M. Ispa, and Duane Rudy. 2006. "Parental Control in Latino Families: An Integrated Review of the Literature." *Child Development* 77 (5):1282–1297.

Hall, Stuart, ed. 1997. *Representation: Cultural Representations and Signifying Practices*. Vol. 2. Sage.

Halperin, Rhoda H. 1998. *Practicing Community: Class Culture and Power in an Urban Neighborhood*. University of Texas Press.

Hanna, Philippe, and Frank Vanclay. 2013. "Human Rights, Indigenous Peoples and the Concept of Free, Prior and Informed Consent." *Impact Assessment and Project Appraisal* 31 (2):146–157.

Hanson, Robert L., Rong Rong, Sayuko Kobes, Yunhua Li Muller, E. Jennifer Weil, Jeffrey M. Curtis, Robert G. Nelson, and Leslie J. Baier. 2015. "The Role of Established Type 2 Diabetes-Susceptibility Genetic Variants in a High-Prevalence American Indian Population." *Diabetes* 64 (7):2646–2657.

Harris, John, ed. 2001. *Bioethics*. Oxford University Press.

Hart, E. Richard. 2018. *American Indian History on Trial: Historical Expertise in Tribal Litigation*. University of Utah Press.

Henrich, Joseph. 2002. "Decision-Making, Cultural Transmission and Adaptation in Economic Anthropology." In *Theory in Economic Anthropology*, edited by J. Ensminger, 251–295. AltaMira Press.

———. 2004. "Cultural Group Selection, Coevolutionary Processes and Large-Scale Cooperation." *Journal of Economic Behavior & Organization* 53 (1):3–35.

Henrich, Joseph, and Richard McElreath. 2007. "Dual-Inheritance Theory: The Evolution of Human Cultural Capacities and Cultural Evolution." In *Oxford Handbook of Evolutionary Psychology*, edited by Robin Ian MacDonald Dunbar, Robin Dunbar, and Louise Barrett, 555–570. Oxford University Press.

Henrich, Natalie, and Joseph Patrick Henrich. 2007. *Why Humans Cooperate: A Cultural and Evolutionary Explanation*. Oxford University Press.

Herzfeld, Michael. 1989. *Anthropology through the Looking-Glass: Critical Ethnography in the Margins of Europe*. Cambridge University Press.

Hilbig, Benjamin E., Isabel Thielmann, Johanna Hepp, Sina A. Klein, and Ingo Zettler. 2015. "From Personality to Altruistic Behavior (and Back): Evidence from a Double-Blind Dictator Game." *Journal of Research in Personality* 55:46–50.

Hill, David. 2018. "Peru Moves to Create Huge New Indigenous Reserves in Peru." *The Guardian*, February 28.

Hindery, Derrick. 2013. *From Enron to Evo: Pipeline Politics, Global Environmentalism, and Indigenous Rights in Bolivia*. University of Arizona Press.

Hodgson, Dorothy L. 2002. "Introduction: Comparative perspectives on the Indigenous Rights Movement in Africa and the Americas." *American Anthropologist* 104 (4): 1037–1049.

Hodžić, Saida. 2009. "Unsettling Power: Domestic Violence, Gender Politics, and Struggles over Sovereignty in Ghana." *Ethnos* 74 (3):331–360.

———. 2013. "Ascertaining Deadly Harms: Aesthetics and Politics of Global Evidence." *Cultural Anthropology* 28 (1):86–109.

———. 2016. *The Twilight of Cutting: African Activism and Life after NGOs*. University of California Press.

Hoeyer, Klaus, and Linda F. Hogle. 2014. "Informed Consent: The Politics of Intent and Practice in Medical Research Ethics." *Annual Review of Anthropology* 43:347–362.

Hofstede, Gert Jan. 2009. "Research on Cultures: How to Use It in Training? " *European Journal of Cross-Cultural Competence and Management* 1 (1): 14–21.

———. 2011. "Dimensionalizing Cultures: The Hofstede Model in Context." *Online Readings in Psychology and Culture* 2 (1). https://doi.org/10.9707/2307-0919.1014.

Hollis, Martin, and Edward J. Nell. 1975. *Rational Economic Man: A Philosophical Critique of Neoclassical Economics*. Cambridge University Press.

Holm, Tom, J. Diane Pearson, and Ben Chavis. 2003. "Peoplehood: A Model for the Extension of Sovereignty in American Indian Studies." *Wicazo Sa Review* 18 (1):7–24.

Horowitz, Carol R., and J. Carey Jackson. 1997. "Female 'Circumcision': African Women Confront American Medicine." *Journal of General Internal Medicine* 12 (8):491–499. doi:10.1046/j.1525-1497.1997.00088.x.

Howard, Heather A. 2018. "Settler Colonial Biogovernance and the Logic of a Surgical Cure for Diabetes." *American Anthropologist* 120 (4): 817–822.

Howard, Heather A., Marsha MacDowell, Judy Pierzynowski, and Laura E. Smith. Forthcoming. "Anishinaabe Makers and the Animation of Material Narratives."

Howard-Bobiwash, Heather.2003. "Women's Class Strategies as Activism in Native Community Building in Toronto, 1950–1975." *American Indian Quarterly* 27 (3): 566–582.

Hoxie, Frederick E. 2008. "Retrieving the Red Continent: Settler Colonialism and the History of American Indians in the US." *Ethnic and Racial Studies* 31 (6): 1153–1167.

Hrdlička, Aleš.1906. "Notes on the Pima of Arizona." *American Anthropologist* 8 (1): 39–46.

Hsu, Francis L. K. 1983. *Rugged Individualism Reconsidered: Essays in Psychological Anthropology.* University of Tennessee Press.

Hsueh, Wen-Chi, Anup K. Nair, Sayuko Kobes, Peng Chen, Harald H. H. Göring, Toni I. Pollin, Alka Malhotra, William C. Knowler, Leslie J. Baier, and Robert L. Hanson. 2017. "Identity-by-Descent Mapping Identifies Major Locus for Serum Triglycerides in Amerindians Largely Explained by an APOC3 Founder Mutation." *Circulation: Genomic and Precision Medicine* 10 (6):e001809.

Hunt, Linda M. 2000. "Strategic Suffering: Illness Narratives as Social Empowerment among Mexican Cancer Patients." In *Narrative and the Cultural Construction of Illness and Healing,* edited by Cheryl Mattingly and Linda Garro, 88–107. University of California-Berkeley.

Humphreys, Michael, and Tony J. Watson. 2009. "Ethnographic practices: From 'Writing-up Ethnographic Research' to 'Writing Ethnography'." In *Organizational Ethnography: Studying the Complexities of Everyday Life,* edited by Sierk Ybema, Dvora Yanow, Harry Wels, and Frans Kamsteed, 40–55. Sage.

Jackson, Jean E., and Kay B. Warren. 2005. "Indigenous Movements in Latin America, 1992–2004: Controversies, Ironies, New Directions." *Annual Review of Anthropology* 34:549–573.

Jadrnak, Jackie. 2006. "Tribes Seek More Research Control." *Albuquerque Journal,* July 7.

Jentoft, Svein, Henry Minde, and Ragnar Nilsen. 2003. *Indigenous Peoples: Resource Management and Global Rights.* Eburon Uitgeverij BV.

Johansen, Bruce Elliott. 1996. *Native American Political Systems and the Evolution of Democracy: An Annotated Bibliography.* Greenwood.

Johnson, Mark. 1994. *Moral Imagination: Implications of Cognitive Science for Ethics.* University of Chicago Press.

Kalberg, Stephen. 1994. "Max Weber's Analysis of the Rise of Monotheism: A Reconstruction." *British Journal of Sociology* 45 (4):563–583.

Kapferer, Bruce. 1976. "Introduction: Transactional Models Reconsidered." In Kapferer, *Transaction and Meaning: Directions in the Anthropology of Exchange and Symbolic Behavior,* 1–22. Institute for the Study of Human Issues.

Kauanui, J. Kēhaulani. 2008. *Hawaiian Blood: Colonialism and the Politics of Sovereignty and Indigeneity.* Duke University Press.

———. 2017. "Sovereignty: An Introduction." *Cultural Anthropology* 32 (3):323–329.

Kawachi, Ichiro, Sankaran Venkata Subramanian, and Daniel Kim. 2008. "Social Capital and Health." In Kawachi, Subramanian, and Kim, *Social Capital and Health,* 1–26. Springer.

Keating, Neal B. 2007. "UN General Assembly Adopts Declaration on the Rights of Indigenous Peoples." *Anthropology News* 48 (8):22–23.

Keed, Rita. 1985. *Memories of Bulgandramine Mission*. Self published.

Kennell, James Leslie. 2011. *The Senses and Suffering: Medical Knowledge, Spirit Possession, and Vaccination Programs in Aja*. Southern Methodist University.

Kenrick, Justin, and Jerome Lewis. 2004. "Indigenous Peoples' Rights and the Politics of the Term 'Indigenous.'" *Anthropology Today* 20 (2):4–9.

Kierans, Ciara. 2015. "Biopolitics and Capital: Poverty, Mobility and the Body-in-Transplantation in Mexico." *Body & Society* 21 (3):42–65.

Kierkegaard, Søren. 1996. *Papers and Journals: A Selection*. Penguin.

Kingsbury, B. 1998. "'Indigenous Peoples' in International Law: A Constructivist Approach to the Asian Controversy." *American Journal of International Law* 92 (3): 414–457.

Kleinman, Arthur. 1976. "Culture, Illness and Care: Clinical Lessons from Anthropologic and Cross-Cultural Research." *Annals of Internal Medicine* 88:251–258.

Kleinman, Arthur. 1980. *Patients and Healers in the Context of Culture: An Exploration of the Borderland between Anthropology, Medicine, and Psychiatry*. Vol. 3. University of California Press.

———. 1999. "Experience and Its Moral Modes: Culture, Human Conditions, and Disorder." *Tanner Lectures on Human Values* 20:355–420.

Konner, Melvin. 1987. *Becoming a Doctor: A Journey of Initiation in Medical School*. Viking.

Kovach, Margaret. 2015. "Emerging from the Margins: Indigenous Methodologies." In *Research as Resistance: Revisiting Critical, Indigenous, and Anti-oppressive Approaches*, edited by Leslie Brown and Susan Strega, 43–64. Canadian Scholars Press.

Kozak, David L. 1997. "Surrendering to Diabetes: An Embodied Response to Perceptions of Diabetes and Death in the Gila River Indian Community." *OMEGA-Journal of Death and Dying* 35 (4):347–359.

Kozak, David L., and David I. Lopez. 1999. *Devil Sickness and Devil Songs: Tohono O'odham Poetics*. Smithsonian Institution Press.

Krech, Shepard. 1999. *The Ecological Indian: Myth and History*. WW Norton & Company.

Krmpotich, Cara, Heather Howard, and Emma Knight. 2016. "From Collection to Community to Collections Again: Urban Indigenous Women, Material Culture and Belonging." *Journal of Material Culture* 21 (3): 343–365.

Kroeber, Alfred Louis, and Clyde Kluckhohn. 1952. "Culture: A Critical Review of Concepts and Definitions." Peabody Museum of Archaeology & Ethnology, Harvard University.

Kuczewski, Mark G. 1999. *Fragmentation and Consensus: Communitarian and Casuist Bioethics*. Georgetown University Press.

———. 2009. "The Common Morality in Communitarian Thought: Reflective Consensus in Public Policy." *Theoretical Medicine and Bioethics* 30 (1):45–54.

Kuper, Adam, Keiichi Omura, Evie Plaice, Alcida Rita Ramos, Steven Robins, and James Suzman. 2003. "The Return of the Native." *Current Anthropology* 44 (3):389–402.

Kusserow, Adrie Suzanne. 1999. "De-homogenizing American Individualism: Socializing Hard and Soft Individualism in Manhattan and Queens." *Ethos* 27 (2):210–234.

———. 2004. *American Individualisms: Child Rearing and Social Class in Three Neighborhoods*. Palgrave Macmillan.

Lacan, Jacques. 1968. "The Mirror-Phase as Formative of the Function of the I." *New Left Review* 51: 71.

La Fontaine, Jean S. 1985. "Person and Individual: Some Anthropological Reflections." In *The Category of the Person: Anthropology, Philosophy, History*, edited by Michael Carrithers, Steven Collines, and Steven Lukes, 123–140. Cambridge University Press.

Lee, Richard Borshay. 2006. "Twenty-first Century Indigenism." *Anthropological Theory* 6 (4): 455–479.

Lewis, Hope. 1995. "Between Irua and Female Genital Mutilation: Feminist Human Rights Discourse and the Cultural Divide." *Harvard Law School Human Rights Journal* 8:1–56.

Li, Tania Murray. 2000. "Locating Indigenous Environmental Knowledge in Indonesia." In *Indigenous Enviromental Knowledge and Its Transformations: Critical Anthropological Perspectives*, edited by Roy Ellen, Peter Parkes, and Alan Bicker, 121–149. Harwood Academic Publisher.

Lightfoot, Sheryl. 2016. *Global Indigenous Politics: A Subtle Revolution*. Routledge.

LiPuma, Edward. 1998. "Modernity and Forms of Personhood in Melanesia." In *Bodies and Persons: Comparative Perspectives from Africa and Melanesia*, edited by Michael Lambek and Andrew Strathern, 53–79. Cambridge University Press.

Lomawaima, K. T., and T. L. McCarty. 2006. *"To Remain Indian": Lessons in Democracy from a Century of Native American Education*. Teachers College Press.

Loure, Edward, and Fred Nelson. 2016. "The Global Land Rights Struggle Is Intensifying." *Guardian*, April 27.

Lovell, Nadia. 1998. *Locality and Belonging*. Psychology Press.

Low, Setha M. 2003. *The Anthropology of Space and Place*. Blackwell.

Macdonald, Gaynor. 2000. "Economies and Personhood: Demand Sharing among the Wiradjuri of New South Wales." *Senri Ethnological Studies* 53:87–111.

———. 2002. "The Struggle for Recognition: A Native Title Story from Peak Hill, New South Wales." *Australian Aboriginal Studies* 1: 87–90.

———. 2004. *Two Steps Forward, Three Steps Back: A Wiradjuri Land Rights Journey: Letters to the Wiradjuri Regional Aboriginal Land Council on Its 20th Anniversary, 1983–2003*. LhR Press.

———. 2005. "Contradictory Visions: The Closure of Bulgandramine Mission." In *Contesting Assimilation*, edited by Tim Rowse and Richard Nile, 187–200. API Network.

———. 2017. "'Promise Me You'll Come to My Funeral': Putting a Value on Wiradjuri Life Through Death." In *Mortality, Mourning and Mortuary Practices in Indigenous Australia*, edited by Katie Glaskin, Myrna Tonkinson, Yasmine Musharbash, and Victoria Burbank, 143–158. Routledge.

———. 2018. "The Role of Allocative Power and Its Diminution in the Constitution and Violation of Wiradjuri Personhood." In *People and Change in Indigenous Australia*, edited by Diane J Austin-Broos and Francesca Merlan, eds., 97–114. University of Hawai'i Press.

———. Forthcoming. *The Wiradjuri Allocative Economy: Racism and Erasure in Australian Anthropology and Policy*.

Macpherson, Crawford Brough, and Frank Cunningham. 1962. *The Political Theory of Possessive Individualism: Hobbes to Locke*. Clarendon Press.

Malkki, Liisa. 1992. "National Geographic: The Rooting of Peoples and the Territorialization of National Identity among Scholars and Refugees." *Cultural Anthropology* 7 (1):24–44.

Manderson, Lenore. 2010. "Social Capital and Inclusion: Locating Wellbeing in Community." *Australian Cultural History* 28 (2–3):233–252.

Marriott, McKim. 1976. "Interpreting Indian Society: A Monistic Alternative to Dumont's Dualism." *Journal of Asian Studies* 36 (1):189–195.

Martinez, David. 2009. *Dakota Philosopher: Charles Eastman and American Indian Thought.* Minnesota Historical Society.

Mattingly, Cheryl. 2014. *Moral Laboratories: Family Peril and the Struggle for a Good Life.* University of California Press.

Mauss, Marcel. [1938] 1985. "A Category of the Human Mind: The Notion of Person; the Notion of Self." In *The Category of the Person: Anthropology, Philosophy, History,* edited by Steven Collines and Steven Lukes, 1–25. Cambridge University Press.

McIvor, Greg. 2018. "Oil Pipelines Can Be Positive for Indigenous People. Here's how." *The Guardian,* June 19.

Mead, Aroha. 2002. "Understanding Maori Intellectual Property Rights." The Inaugural Maori Legal Forum, available at: www. conferenz. co. nz/library/m/mead_aroha. html.

Merry, Sally Engle. 2003. "Human Rights Law and the Demonization of Culture (and Anthropology along the Way)." *Polar: Political and Legal Anthropology Review* 26 (1): 55–76.

Michielutte, Robert, Penny C. Sharp, Mark B. Dignan, and Karen Blinson. 1994. "Cultural Issues in the Development of Cancer Control Programs for American Indian." *Journal of Health Care for the Poor and Underserved* 5 (4):280–296.

Minde, H., ed. 2008. *Indigenous Peoples: Self-Determination, Knowledge, Indigeneity.* Eburon.

Moemeka, Andrew A. 1998. "Communalism as a Fundamental Dimension of Culture." *Journal of Communication* 48 (4):118–141.

Mohanram, Radhika. 1999. *Black Body: Women, Colonialism, and Space.* Vol. 6. University of Minnesota Press.

Mol, Annemarie. 2008. *The Logic of Care: Health and the Problem of Patient Choice.* Routledge.

Mol, Annemarie, Ingunn Moser, and Jeannette Pols, eds. 2015. *Care in Practice: On Tinkering in Clinics, Homes and Farms.* Transcript Verlag.

Moreton-Robinson, Aileen, ed. 2007. *Sovereign Subjects: Indigenous Sovereignty Matters.* Allen & Unwin.

———. 2011. "Virtuous Racial States: The Possessive Logic of Patriarchal White Sovereignty and the United Nations Declaration on the Rights of Indigenous Peoples." *Griffith Law Review* 20 (3):641–658.

———. 2015. *The White Possessive: Property, Power, and Indigenous Sovereignty.* University of Minnesota Press.

Morgan, Rhiannon. 2007. "On Political Institutions and Social Movement Dynamics: The Case of the United Nations and the Global Indigenous Movement." *International Political Science Review* 28 (3):273–292.

Moser, Caroline O. N. 2004. *Urban Violence and Insecurity: An Introductory Roadmap.* Sage.

Mosse, David. 1997. "The Symbolic Making of a Common Property Resource: History, Ecology and Locality in a Tank-Irrigated Landscape in South India." *Development and Change* 28 (3):467–504.

———. 1999. "Colonial and Contemporary Ideologies of 'Community Management': The Case of Tank Irrigation Development in South India." *Modern Asian Studies* 33 (2):303–338.

———. 2006. "Collective Action, Common Property, and Social Capital in South India: An Anthropological Commentary." *Economic Development and Cultural Change* 54 (3):695–724.

Muehlebach, Andrea. 2001. "'Making Place' at the United Nations: Indigenous Cultural Politics at the UN Working Group on Indigenous Populations." *Cultural Anthropology* 16 (3):415–448.

———. 2003. "What Self in Self-Determination? Notes from the Frontiers of Transnational Indigenous Activism." *Identities* 10 (2): 241–268.

Murphy, Michael A. 2008. "Representing Indigenous Self-Determination." *University of Toronto Law Journal* 58 (2):185–216.

Nabokov, Isabelle. 2000. *Religion against the Self: An Ethnography of Tamil rituals.* Oxford University Press.

Neel, James V. 1962. "Diabetes Mellitus: A 'Thrifty' Genotype Rendered Detrimental by 'Progress'?" *American Journal of Human Genetics* 14 (4):353–362.

Newman, Peter A. 2006. "Towards a Science of Community Engagement." *The Lancet* 367 (9507): 302.

Ngoitiko, Maanda, and Fred Nelson. 2013. "What Africa Can Learn from Tanzania's Remarkable Masai Land Rights Victory." *Guardian*, October 8.

Nnamuchi, Obiajulu. 2018. "Commodification of Body Parts and Its Apologetics: What Is the Position of Human Rights?" *Human Rights Quarterly* 40 (1):168–193.

Novo, Carmen Martínez. 2006. *Who Defines Indigenous?: Identities, Development, Intellectuals, and the State in Northern Mexico.* Rutgers University Press.

Nygren, Anja.1999. "Local Knowledge in the Environment–Development Discourse: From Dichotomies to Situated Knowledges." *Critique of Anthropology* 19 (3): 267–288.

Ohnuki-Tierney, Emiko. 1984. *Illness and Culture in Contemporary Japan: An Anthropological View.* Cambridge University Press.

Oldham, Paul, and Miriam Anne Frank. 2008. "'We the Peoples . . .': The United Nations Declaration on the Rights of Indigenous Peoples." *Anthropology Today* 24 (2):5–9.

Orange, Tommy. 2018. *There, There.* Knopf.

Orenstein, Peggy. 2010. "I Tweet, Therefore I Am." *New York Times*, July 30.

Overing, Joanna, and Alan Passes. 2002. *The Anthropology of Love and Anger: The Aesthetics of Conviviality in Native Amazonia.* Routledge.

Parezo, Nancy J. 1993. *Hidden Scholars: Women Anthropologists and the Native American Southwest.* University of New Mexico Press.

Petryna, Adriana, Andrew Lakoff, and Arthur Kleinman, eds. 2006. *Global Pharmaceuticals: Ethics, Markets, Practices.* Duke University Press.

Piquemal, Nathalie. 2001. "Free and Informed Consent in Research Involving Native American Communities." *American Indian Culture and Research Journal* 25 (1):65–79.

Pitkin, Hanna Fenichel, ed.1969. *Representation.* Atherton Press.

Portes, Alejandro. 1998. "Social Capital: Its Origins and Applications in Modern Sociology." *Annual Review of Sociology* 24 (1):1–24.

Powell, Evelyn, and Gaynor Marilyn Macdonald. 2001. *Keeping That Good Name: How Fred Powell of the Bogan River Wiradjuri Built a Cultural Bridge.* Let Her Rip Press.

Powell, Malea. 2002. "Rhetorics of Survivance: How American Indians Use Writing." *College Composition and Communication* 53 (3): 96–434.

Putnam, Robert D. 2001. *Bowling Alone: The Collapse and Revival of American Community.* Simon and Schuster.

Quesada, James, Laurie Kain Hart, and Philippe Bourgois. 2011. "Structural Vulnerability and Health: Latino Migrant Laborers in the United States." *Medical Anthropology* 30 (4):339–362.

Ragavan, Srividhya. 2001. "Protection of Traditional Knowledge." *Minnesota Intellectual Property Law Review* 2 (2): 1–60

Raibmon, Paige. 2005. "'Handicapped by Distance and Transportation': Indigenous Relocation, Modernity and Time-Space Expansion." *American Studies* 46 (3–4): 363–390.

———. 2007. "Meanings of Mobility on the Northwest Coast." In *New Histories for Old: Changing Perspectives on Canada's Native Pasts*, edited by Ted Binnema and Susan Neylan, 175–195. University of Washington Press.

———. 2008. "Unmaking Native Space: A Genealogy of Indian Policy, Settler Practice, and the Microtechniques of Dispossession." In *The Power of Promises: Rethinking Indian Treaties in the Pacific Northwest*, edited by Alexandra Harmon, 56–85. University of Washington Press.

Ramirez, Renya K. 2007. *Native Hubs: Culture, Community, and Belonging in Silicon Valley and Beyond*. Duke University Press.

Ramos, Alcida R. 1987. "Reflecting on the Yanomami: Ethnographic Images and the Pursuit of the Exotic." *Cultural Anthropology* 2 (3):284–304.

———. 1994. "The Hyperreal Indian." *Critique of Anthropology* 14 (2):153–171.

———. 1998. *Indigenism: Ethnic Politics in Brazil*. University of Wisconsin Press.

Rapport, Nigel. 1997. *Transcendent Individual*. Taylor & Francis.

———. 1998. "Time with the Other: A Diary in the AAA Sense of the Term." *Anthropology Today* 14 (1): 19–21.

———. 2002. *Transcendent Individual: Essays Toward a Literary and Liberal Anthropology*. Routledge.

———. 2012. "The Politics of Perspectivism." *Annual Review of Anthropology* 41: 481–494.

Rawls, John. 2009. *A Theory of Justice*. Rev. ed. Harvard University Press.

Rea, Amadeo M. 1997. *At the Desert's Green Edge: An Ethnobotany of the Gila River Pima*. University of Arizona Press.

Rimmer, Matthew, ed. 2015. *Indigenous Intellectual Property: A Handbook of Contemporary Research*: Edward Elgar.

Robert, General Henry M. 1921. *Robert's Rules of Order Revised*. Da Capo Press.

Rodman, Margaret C. 1992. "Empowering Place: Multilocality and Multivocality." *American Anthropologist* 94 (3):640–656.

Rostosky, Sharon Scales, and Cheryl Brown Travis. 1996. "Menopause Research and the Dominance of the Biomedical Model 1984–1994." *Psychology of Women Quarterly* 20 (2):285–312.

Roth, Christopher F. 2002. "Goods, Names, and Selves: Rethinking the Tsimshian Potlatch." *American Ethnologist* 29 (1):123–150.

Rousseau, Jean-Jacques. [1762] 1978. *On the Social Contract*. Edited by Roger D. Masters. Translated by Judith R. Masters. St. Martin's.

Russell, Frank. 1903. "Pima Annals." *American Anthropologist* 5 (1): 76–80.

———. 1908. *The Pima Indians*. Bureau of American Ethnology.

Sahota, Puneet Chawla. 2012. "Genetic Histories: Native Americans' Accounts of Being at Risk for Diabetes." *Social Studies of Science* 42 (6):821–842.

Sand, Sabine. 2002. "Sui Generis Laws for the Protection of Indigenous Expressions of Culture and Traditional Knowledge." *University of Queensland Law Journal* 22: 188–198.

Sandberg, Sveinung. 2008. "Street Capital: Ethnicity and Violence on the Streets of Oslo." *Theoretical Criminology* 12 (2): 153–171.

Sargent, Carolyn, and Carolyn Smith-Morris. 2006. "Questioning Our Principles: Anthropological Contributions to Ethical Dilemmas in Clinical Practice." *Cambridge Quarterly of Healthcare Ethics* 15 (2):123–134.

Saugestad, Sidsel. 2001. *The Inconvenient Indigenous: Remote Area Development in Botswana, Donor Assistance and the First People of the Kalahari*. Nordic Africa Institute.

———. 2011. "Impact of International Mechanisms on Indigenous Rights in Botswana." *International Journal of Human Rights* 15 (1):37–61.

Sawyer, Suzana, and Edmund Terence Gomez. 2012. *The Politics of Resource Extraction: Indigenous Peoples, Multinational Corporations and the State*. Palgrave Macmillan.

Schroedel, Jean Reith, and Artour Aslanian. 2017. "A Case Study of Descriptive Representation: The Experience of Native American Elected Officials in South Dakota." *American Indian Quarterly* 41 (3):250–286.

Schwartzman, Stephan, and Barbara Zimmerman. 2005. "Conservation Alliances with Indigenous Peoples of the Amazon." *Conservation Biology* 19 (3):721–727.

Scott, Craig. 1996. "Indigenous Self-Determination and Decolonization of the International Imagination: A Plea." *Human Rights Quarterly* 18 (4):814–820.

Scott, James C. 1985. *Weapons of the Weak: Everyday Forms of Peasant Resistance*. Yale University Press.

Sengupta, Roshni. 2005. "Communal Violence in India: Perspectives on Causative Factors." *Economic and Political Weekly* 40 (20): 2046–2050.

Service, Elman Rogers. 1971. *Primitive Social Organization: An Evolutionary Perspective*. Random House.

Shaw, Anna Moore. 2016. *A Pima Past*. University of Arizona Press.

Shell-Duncan, Bettina, and Ylva Hernlund. 2000. *Female "Circumcision" in Africa: Culture, Controversy, and Change*. Lynne Rienner.

Sieder, Rachel, and Anna Barrera. 2017. "Women and Legal Pluralism: Lessons from Indigenous Governance Systems in the Andes." *Journal of Latin American Studies* 49 (3): 633–658.

Singh, Pritam. 2015. "Institutional Communalism in India." *Economic and Political Weekly* 50 (28):48–56.

Sium, Aman, Chandni Desai, and Eric Ritskes. 2012. "Towards the 'tangible Unknown': Decolonization and the Indigenous Future." *Decolonization: Indigeneity, Education & Society* 1 (1): I-XIII

Smith-Morris, Carolyn M. 2004. "Reducing Diabetes in Indian Country: Lessons from the Three Domains Influencing Pima Diabetes." *Human Organization* 63 (1):34–46.

———. 2005. "Diagnostic Controversy: Gestational Diabetes and the Meaning of Risk for Pima Indian Women." *Medical Anthropology* 24 (2):145–177.

———. 2006a. "Community Participation in Tribal Diabetes Programming." *American Indian Culture & Research Journal* 30 (2):85–110.

———. 2006b. *Diabetes among the Pima: Stories of Survival*. University of Arizona Press.

———. 2007. "Autonomous Individuals or Self-Determined Communities? The Changing Ethics of Research among Native Americans." *Human Organization* 66 (3):327–336.

———. 2008. "Social Capital in a Mexican American Community in Dallas, Texas." *Urban Anthropology* 36 (4):1–32.

———. 2016. "The Traditional Food of Migrants: Meat, Water, and Other Challenges for Dietary Advice. An Ethnography in Guanajuato, Mexico." *Appetite* 105:430–438.

———. 2017. "Epidemiological Placism in Public Health Emergencies: Ebola in Two Dallas Neighborhoods." *Social Science & Medicine* 179:106–114.

Smith-Morris, Carolyn, and Jenny Epstein. 2014. "Beyond Cultural Competency: Skill, Reflexivity, and Structure in Successful Tribal Health Care." *American Indian Culture & Research Journal* 38 (1): 29–48.

Smith-Morris, Carolyn, Daisy Morales-Campos, Edith Alejandra Cataneda Alvarez, and Matthew Turner. 2013. "An Anthropology of *Familismo*: On Narratives and Description of Mexican/Immigrants." *Hispanic Journal of Behavioral Sciences* 35 (1): 35–60.

Snead, James E., Clark L. Erickson, and J. Andrew Darling. 2011. *Landscapes of Movement: Trails, Paths, and Roads in Anthropological Perspective.* University of Pennsylvania Press.

Spiro, Melford E. 1956. *Kibbutz: Venture in Utopia.* Harvard university Press.

———. 1958. *Children of the Kibbutz.* Harvard university Press.

Stack, Carol B. 1975. *All Our Kin: Strategies for Survival in a Black Community.* Basic Books.

Steelman, Toddi A., Lindy Coejuell, Christina Cromley, and Christine Edwards. 2013. *Adaptive Governance: Integrating Science, Policy, and Decision Making.* Columbia University Press.

Stewart-Harawira, Makere. 2005. *The New Imperial Order: Indigenous Responses to Globalization.* Zed Books.

Stoller, Paul. 1984. "Sound in Songhay Cultural Experience." *American Ethnologist* 11 (3):559–570.

Strathern, Marilyn. 1988. *The Gender of the Gift: Problems with Women and Problems with Society in Melanesia.* University of California Press.

———. 2004. "The Whole Person and Its Artifacts." *Annual Review of Anthropology* 33:1–19.

———. 2005. *Partial Connections.* Rowman Altamira.

Stromberg, Ernest, ed. 2006a. *American Indian Rhetorics of Survivance: Word Medicine, Word Magic.* University of Pittsburgh Press.

———. 2006b. "Resistance and Mediation: The Rhetoric of Irony in Indian Boarding School Narratives by Francis La Flesche and Zitkala-Sa." In Stromberg, *American Indian Rhetorics of Survivance,* 95–109.

Sutton, Peter. 2004. *Native Title in Australia: An Ethnographic Perspective.* Cambridge University Press.

———. 2009. *The Politics of Suffering: Indigenous Australia and the End of the Liberal Consensus.* Melbourne University Publishing.

Sykes, Karen. 2009. "Residence: Moral Reasoning in a Common Place—Paradoxes of a Global Age." In *Ethnographies of Moral Reasoning,* 3–40. Springer.

———. 2012. "Moral Reasoning." In *A Companion to Moral Anthropology,* edited by Didier Fassin, 169–185. John Wiley.

Sylvain, Renée. 2014. "Essentialism and the Indigenous Politics of Recognition in Southern Africa." *American Anthropologist* 116 (2): 251–264.

Szreter, Simon, and Michael Woolcock. 2004. "Health by Association? Social Capital, Social Theory, and the Political Economy of Public Health." *International Journal of Epidemiology* 33 (4):650–667.

Thompson, Richard H. 1997. "Ethnic Minorities and the Case for Collective Rights." *American Anthropologist* 99 (4):786–798.

Thornton, Russell. 1990. *American Indian Holocaust and Survival: A Population History since 1492.* Vol. 186. University of Oklahoma Press.

Treuer, David. 2012. *Rez Life: An Indian's Journey through Reservation Life.* Grove/ Atlantic.

Turner, Victor. 1969. "Liminality and Communitas." In Turner, *The Ritual Process: Structure and Anti-structure,* 94–130. Routledge.

Underhill, Ruth Murray. 1936. *The Autobiography of a Papago Woman.* American Anthropological Association.

———. 1985. *Papago Woman.* Waveland Press.

———. 2000. *The Papapo (Tohono O'odham) and Pima Indians of Arizona.* Filter Press.

Underhill, Ruth, and Velino Herrera. [1941] 2000. *The Papago (Tohono O'Odham) and Pima Indians of Arizona.* Filter Press.

Venkateswar, Sita, and Emma Hughes, eds. 2011. *The Politics of Indigeneity: Dialogues and Reflections on Indigenous Activism.* Zed Books.

Verran, Helen. 1998. "Re-imagining Land Ownership in Australia." *Postcolonial Studies* 1 (2):237–254.

Vertovec, Steven. 2007. "Super-diversity and Its Implications." *Ethnic & Racial Studies* 30 (6):1024–1054.

———. 2013. "Reading Super-diversity." www.mmg.mpg.de.

Vidal, John. 2016. "The Tribes Paying the Brutal Price of Conservation" *The Guardian,* August 28.

Wade, Derick T., and Peter W. Halligan. 2004. "Do Biomedical Models of Illness Make for Good Healthcare Systems?" *BMJ* 329 (7479):1398–1401.

Wailoo, Keith, and Stephen Pemberton. 2006. *The Troubled Dream of Genetic Medicine: Ethnicity and Innovation in Tay-Sachs, Cystic Fibrosis, and Sickle Cell Disease.* Johns Hopkins University Press.

Waitere, Hine, and Elizabeth Allen. 2011. "Beyond Indigenous Civilities: Indigenous Matters." In Venkateswar and Hughes, *The Politics of Indigeneity: Dialogues and Reflections on Indigenous Activism,* 45–74.

Wallerstein, Nina B., and Bonnie Duran. 2006. "Using Community-Based Participatory Research to Address Health Disparities." *Health Promotion Practice* 7 (3):312–323.

Wax, Murray L. 1991. "The Ethics of Research in American Indian Communities." *American Indian Quarterly* 15 (4): 431–456.

Waziyatawin, Angela, and M. Yellow Bird, eds. 2012. *For Indigenous Minds Only: A Decolonization Handbook.* School of American Research Press.

Werbner, Richard. 2002. "Conclusion: Citizenship and the Politics of Recognition in Botswana." In *Minorities in the Millennium: Perspectives from Botswana, edited by* Isaac N. Mazonde, 117–135. Lightbooks.

Wickham, Molly. 2012. "Initiating the Process of Youth Decolonization: Reclaiming Our Right to Know and Act on Our Experiences." In Waziyatawin and Yellow Bird, *For Indigenous Minds Only,* 179–203.

Wiedman, D. 2010. Globalizing the chronicities of modernity: Diabetes and the metabolic syndrome. In *Chronic Conditions, Fluid States: Chronicity and the Anthropology of Illness,* edited by Lenore Manderson and Carolyn Smith-Morris. Rutgers University Press.

———. 2012. "Native American Embodiment of the Chronicities of Modernity: Reservation Food, Diabetes, and the Metabolic Syndrome among the Kiowa, Comanche, and Apache." *Medical Anthropology Quarterly* 26 (4): 595–612.

Wilkie, Meredith. 1985. *Aboriginal Land Rights in NSW.* Alternative Publishing Co-op.

Wissler, Clark. 1927. "The Culture-Area Concept in Social Anthropology." *American Journal of Sociology* 32 (6): 881–891.

Wolf, Eric R. 1982. *Europe and the People without History.* University of California Press.

Wolfe, Patrick. 1991. "On Being Woken Up: The Dreamtime in Anthropology and in Australian Settler Culture." *Comparative Studies in Society and History* 33 (2):197–224.

Woolcock, Geoffrey, and Lenore Manderson. 2009. *Social Capital and Social Justice: Critical Australian Perspectives.* Charles Darwin University Press.

Woolcock, Michael, and Deepa Narayan. 2000. "Social Capital: Implications for Development Theory, Research, and Policy." *World Bank Research Observer* 15 (2):225–249.

Wynn, Julia, and Wendy K. Chung. 2017. "23andMe Paves the Way for Direct-to-Consumer Genetic Health Risk Tests of Limited Clinical Utility." *Annals of Internal Medicine* 167 (2):125–126.

Yates-Doerr, Emily. 2012. "The Weight of the Self: Care and Compassion in Guatemalan Dietary Choices." *Medical Anthropology Quarterly* 26 (1):136–158.

———. 2015. *The Weight of Obesity: Hunger and Global Health in Postwar Guatemala.* University of California Press.

Youkee, Mat. 2018. "'We Burned the Forest': The Indigenous Chileans Fighting Loggers with Arson." *The Guardian,* June 14.

Young, Allan. 1981. "The Creation of Medical Knowledge: Some Problems in Interpretation." *Social Science & Medicine* 15 (3): 317–335.

Index

academics, 4–7, 12, 20, 23, 40, 106, 125, 137–138
agency, 34, 72, 92
agriculture, 14, 15, 67, 86, 128
Akimel O'odham, xiii, 2, 4, 14–17, 20, 38–39, 73, 141–143 passim. *See also* Pima
"alienable," 69, 73, 75, 119, 139n3
altruism, 4, 29, 36, 96, 103, 119
ancestors, xv, 27, 35, 41, 45; ancestral authority, 40–41; ancestral sites, lands, territories, x–xi, 7–11, 20, 40, 46, 103, 132; ancestral social networks, 131; change to ancestral forms (traditions), 87; invocation of, 27; proper relations with, 69, 72, 103, 124, 127–130
anonymity, 33, 70, 135
applied anthropology, 4, 20, 23, 74, 75, 110, 139n3
Aristotle, 58, 144n4
association, 6, 9, 35, 57, 98, 99, 116, 121, 140n6
Australian Aborigines, ix, 144n5. *See also* Wiradjuri Aborigines
authenticity, 67, 86, 104, 116, 139–140n4
authority: authoritative ideologies of medicine, 113, 114; authority to speak, 27, 28, 31, 92, 116; communal authority, 33; of communities to set rules for members, 90; contests of, 116; hyperindividualist strategies taken as, 110; Indigenous styles of, 59; introductions as link to, 27; legal, 125; in naming practices, 90–91, 97; of nation-state,

133, 146n11; networks of, 33; to officiate/approve/grant search for, 56, 67; place-based forms of, 40; public authority, 34; relational authority, 59; and representation, 68–72; risk of too much authority, 38
autonomy: authority, 56; choice, 57, 104, 114; engagements, 26; Indigenous peoples, 20; individual/personal, 10, 56–57, 81, 91, 104, 106–110; long-term Indigenous, 115, 127; O'odham communities, 6; of the patient, 117, 119; presumption of, 109; seeking one's own, 114, 144n6; threatened, 2.

balance, 22, 49, 63, 70, 75, 88, 101, 105, 131, 133; communal, 3, 10; of communalism and individualism, 2, 11, 18, 43, 92–103, 113, 116, 123, 144n19; of values, 23
belonging, 104; *communitas*, 34; consensus as practice of, 41; as a feature of indigeneity, 2, 134; to land, ix; mark of, 115; as more than membership/membership rules, 42, 54; as one of four elements of communalism, 21–23, 25–44, 86, 106, 120, 124; participation/commitment, 41, 61; and place, 143n16; sense of, 21, 26, 34, 41, 115, 120, 124, 130; touchstones of, 39, 43
binaries, 4, 5, 59, 103, 126
biogovernance, 112. *See also* governance
bloodlines, 26, 78, 99, 146n2; blood-and-soil, 2, 8, 127; blood quantum, 42, 76, 130, 143n18

About the Author

Carolyn Smith-Morris is an associate professor of anthropology at Southern Methodist University in Dallas, Texas. She is the author of *Diabetes among the Pima*, editor of *Diagnostic Controversy: Cultural Perspectives on Competing Knowledge in Healthcare*, and co-editor of *Chronic Conditions, Fluid States: Chronicity and the Anthropology of Illness*.

Printed and bound by CPI Group (UK) Ltd, Croydon, CR0 4YY

16/04/2025

14658333-0001